I0842411

Dementia-Mama-Drama

A Daily Dose of Dementia with Mama Drama

Hopeful, Humorous and Helpful

Vincent Zappacosta

Copyright ©2020
By Vincent Zappacosta
ISBN:9798644596867

All rights reserved. No part of this book may be
reproduced, scanned or distributed in any printed
or electronic form without permission.

Editor: Douglass Christensen
Cover Design and Photography: nyc2vin

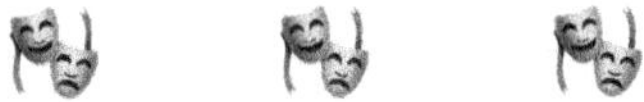

This book is dedicated to caregivers
all over the world
who selflessly devote their time
and who face the daily challenge
of their own "drama".

This year would have been Mama's 100th
birthday. It's the perfect time to share
and celebrate her life.
She taught me that love, music and humor
could get you through anything.

This is for you Mama 

DAILY DOSES

THE "DRAMA" CAST

Son: Vincent
Mama: Anna
Son-in-Law: Douglass

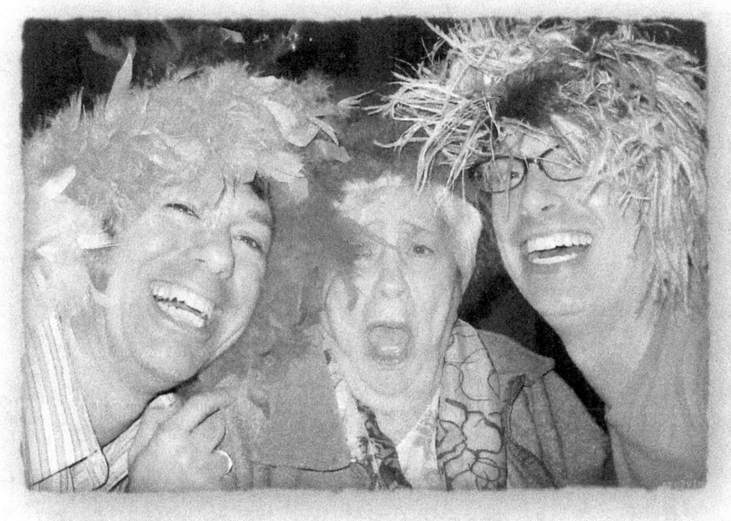

SETTING:
Village Nursing Home, NY
Rafael Nursing Home, CA

TIME:
Fall 2000 thru Winter 2013

Preface

Welcome to the relationship of a modern family... a mother, her son and his husband. Today's family may look different but the feelings are the same as we all begin to switch roles caring for our aging parents. This is our story of the daily doses of dementia with Mama and the bumpy bittersweet ride we shared as caregivers for thirteen years. I want to inspire caregivers and show how being creative and not always following the rules could lead to finding your own way of coping with caregiving. We dealt with it all through the power of humor, music and a lot of love.

Our book began as therapy documenting our daily visits with Mama in our blog, Dementia-Mama-Drama. During that time it became an essential coping tool for all of us. It followed our ups and downs with the disease by sharing how we used humor in a seemingly hopeless situation. I would like caregivers to know it's possible to make lemonade out of lemons, being thankful for what IS rather than what WAS or what WILL BE. Living in the moment while juggling a few hats has its rewards, it did for us.

Mama wanted her story to be told and we promised we would tell it. She loved that we were writing about her. She was excited that people from all over the world were very responsive to our blog. They were connecting with us straight from the heart and the applause was like a boost of energy for Mama. She finally got her moment of fame that she always wanted and she reveled in it.

The book changed again when we were asked to adapt it as a play which was accepted into The Fringe Festival. We continue to develop the play "Some of These Daze" and have had several readings on both coasts.

We know many of you will relate to our "Daily Doses" and they'll bring a smile, a tear or a little hope helping you through your own "Dementia Drama."

Your Mother Is Fine, But...
She Has Dementia

I don't know when I became fully aware of it, but at some point, I became my mother's caregiver. It's not a role I would ever have chosen. I didn't have pets, children or anything else that could make my life more complicated or chaotic, that has always been my choice. But something changed when I no longer had that freedom, it was called dementia.

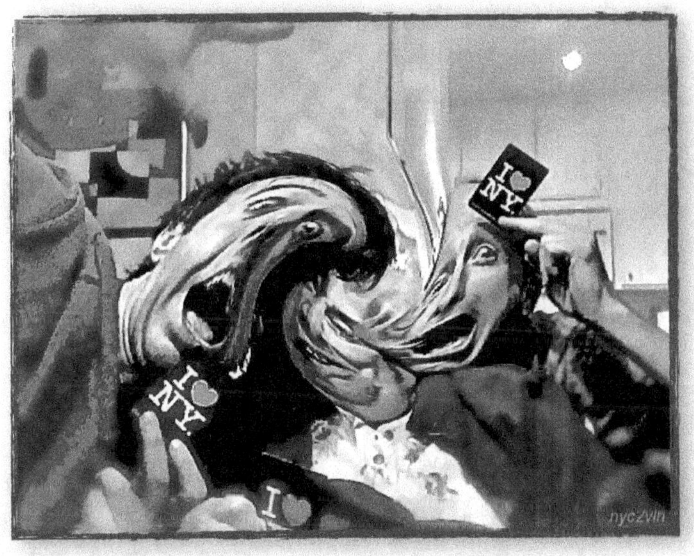

When I first found out my mother was diagnosed with dementia and the onset of Alzheimer's, I didn't know what to do. I just dealt with it, what else could I do? It was what it was, not much was known about this awful disease back then.

It was in the fall of 2000 and I was sitting in the social workers office checking in my mothers clothes admitting her into her first nursing home. I fought very hard to get her in there, it was only one block away from my apartment in NYC. After all I would be checking up on her and the staff everyday. I knew that after being discharged from her short term rehab, she wasn't going to be able to go back home and live on her own ever again. I was scared, the reality was overwhelming and I had to make a lot of big decisions. I was very emotional as I tagged her

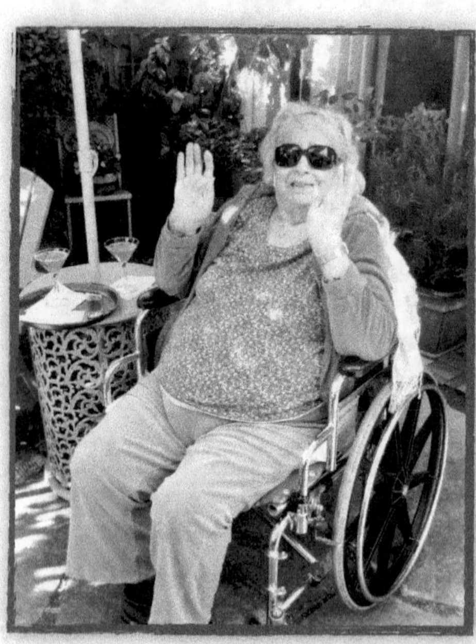

clothes and fought back the tears. My mother was NEVER going into a nursing home - I would not allow it! At least that's what I thought. I continued separating her blouses from her sweaters and slacks as I tried to remain focused. My mother made a remarkable recovery from a high risk surgery. She had a pulmonary embolectomy

as a result of undiagnosed heart disease,
a silent killer in women. The social
worker said "*Your mother is fine, but she
has dementia...*" What? This was the first
time that I heard the word dementia
attached to MY mother. I didn't want to
hear it, I didn't want to believe it. She
knew who I was, she knew how to play cards
and carry on most conversations. Her sense
of humor was still salty and even joked
about her aches and pains. She knew the
words to almost every song and if not, was
somehow able to make the lyrics still
rhyme. So how could it be that my mother
had dementia? Little did I know at the
time that her surgery could have caused
post operative cognitive decline or onset
dementia.

I didn't fully understand what that
meant. I didn't want to believe the
doctors diagnosis, but deep down I knew
something wasn't right. I'm not a doctor,
but learned about the disease by living
with it. I dealt with it the only way I
knew how, by being there, always asking
the doctors questions and constantly being
the squeaky wheel. The way my husband
Douglass and I dealt with it during our
daily visits was by singing, playing
cards, exercising and adding humor at the
most inappropriate moments - that's how WE
did it.

My mother and I always had a very close relationship, we usually "got" each other. She was very supportive and allowed me to be different as a child. But she was also overprotective and neurotic - Anna was an Italian from New York after all! We always spoke our minds and had a very honest and VERY direct way of speaking to each other, okay we yelled and cursed. But the tables turned with dementia. I became "the parent" and Mama "the child," there was a complete role reversal. We had a bond that couldn't be broken and I would not have had it any other way. I became the caregiver because I didn't trust anyone else to do it and there was no one else that knew her like I did. I didn't realize it at the time, but that was the beginning of my life as a caregiver.

I knew Mama loved to sing and be on camera, so we started recording videos during our daily visits. We shared many of them on *YouTube* and our blog, *Dementia-Mama-Drama*. We discovered that music would make her come alive and she loved the attention, I think we created a monster. Sometimes she'd break into song just to change the subject or because she forgot the answer to a question. She was one helluva singer. Music is a very powerful tool and thankfully it changed her mood and ours.

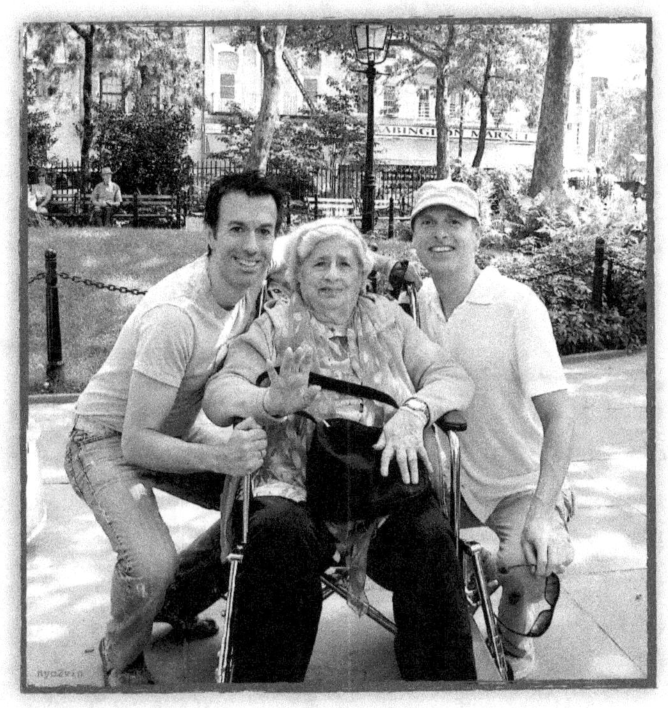

We decided to share our experiences as caregivers and hopefully help others. I know many of you will recognize some of them and realize that you are NOT alone.

Mama's Macaroni

Food was everything to Mama, she loved her food. Truth be told, she was obsessed with food up until the end. She was always *starving* and wanted to eat. Some of Mama's most vivid memories that Alzheimer's couldn't erase were of food.

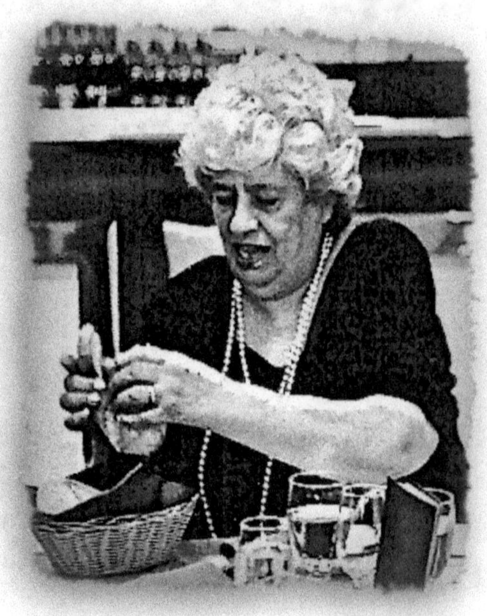

Growing up in an Italian family, pasta was always the main event. Everything else was secondary, especially to Mama. Years later whenever holidays were near, we'd ask her what she wanted to have for dinner. It didn't matter if it was Easter, Thanksgiving, Christmas or her birthday, it was always the same answer. She wanted macaroni, gravy and maybe a meatball. She would *never* say pasta, it was always macaroni, just like it was always gravy, *never* sauce. I tried explaining the difference to her many times, but old habits die hard.

    Whenever Mama would come over for
dinner, we'd have the same conversation
about planning the menu. The difference
was that now there were only the three of
us and she wasn't doing the cooking...

Vin: Mama, what do you want to eat when
you come over tomorrow?

Mama: What the hell do you think I wanna
eat? What do I always wanna eat?

Douglass: Pasta?

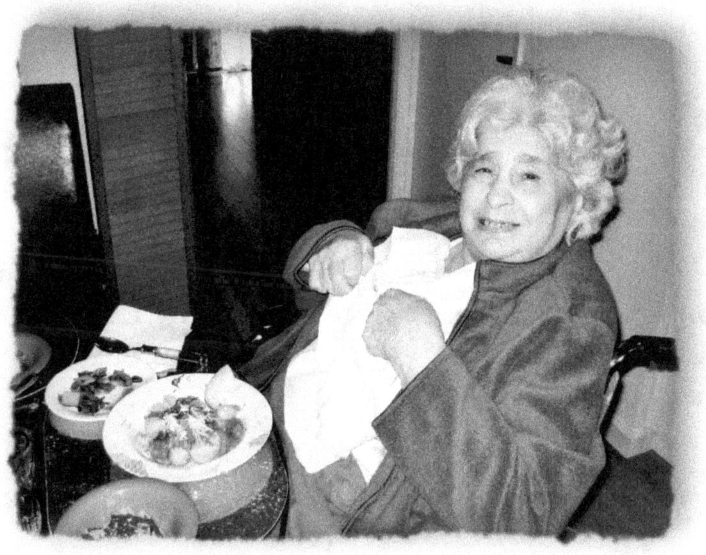

Mama: Of course, what's wrong with you? I
want my spaghetti and meatballs or any
kind of macaroni. My mouth is watering
just thinking about it. Ohhh my God, now
I'm starving.

Vin: Okay Ma, we'll make your favorite dish as usual, as long as that'll make you happy.

Mama: I'm coming over to your place, right?

Douglass: Yes, you're coming over to our place.

Mama: Then that'll make me happy. Just make sure we have some macaroni with lots of cheese and some good Italian bread.

Vin: Okay, okay. Anything else?

Mama: Yeah, don't forget the coffee and cake. Oh my God, I'm gonna dream about it all night!

Food *was* everything to Mama. The next day she was loving her macaroni and gravy as Douglass and I were enjoying our pasta and sauce.

I Have No Options

Before dementia and before cell phones, Mama understood the concept of answering machines... almost. She would call and leave a message going on as though she was actually talking to me - sighing, cursing, asking questions and ending with "Call me right away." Fast forward to when she had the nurses call me on my cell phone from the nursing home. They'd call my cell phone and when I wasn't able to pick up the phone, my message came on just like an answering machine and they'd hand her the phone...

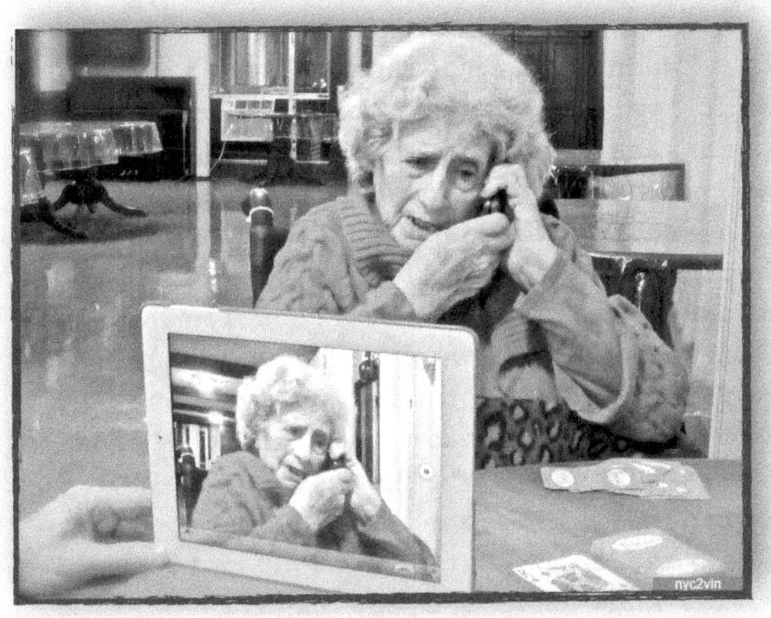

The message that Mama usually left was: "Hello, hello, HELLOOOOO. Nurse, nurse, something is wrong with this phone. No one is answering, can you dial my son Vincent again?" *(Click)*

A few minutes later another call and another message: "Hello, hello, HELLOOOOO. Oh damn it, no one is there. Nurse, this phone is NOT working. You must have the wrong number. No one knows what they are doing in this damn place. Hello, nurse, I don't know what's wrong. Can you please hang this phone up for me? No one is answering. Hellooooo Nurse... NURSE can you pleeease hang up this damn phone? Ohhh, Mother of God!" *(Click)*

When I visited her later that day, I went over the basic mechanics of the cell phone again and explained it's just like an answering machine. I let her hear my pre-recorded message and told her when you hear *my* message end, then you leave *your* message and *not* scream... "Hello, hello, HELLOOOOO." It's a recorded message, I'm NOT there, I can't pick up my phone. My pre-recorded message ends with "Please leave a message at the beep or select your options." She looked at me shaking her head and said "But I have no options." And I knew that she was right.

Does It Really Matter?

It happens to me more and more on a
daily basis. I remember the past and think
of it like it was yesterday. It's hard to
believe how much time has passed since
certain events have happened in my life.
It seems like
yesterday that I
was a fat frenetic
five year old kid
that sang along to
his Judy Garland
albums. It seems
like only yesterday
that I graduated
from high school.
And it seems just
like yesterday that
I was moving into
my very first
apartment.

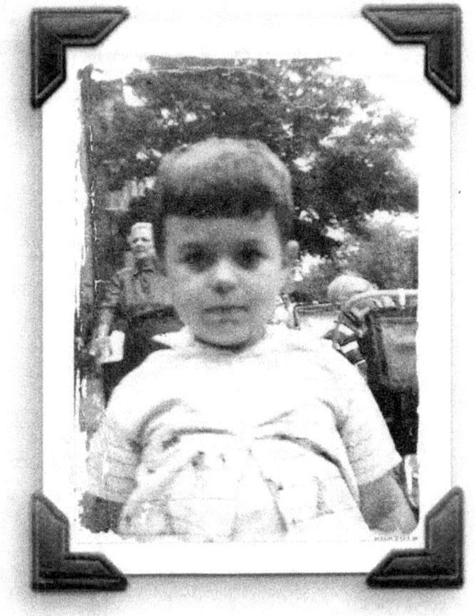

Time gets confusing for all of us,
but imagine what it's like for someone
with dementia or Alzheimer's. I tried to
put myself in my mother's place. I tried
to think what does *she* really remember?
What is *her* time frame? I often asked her
questions to check in with her, keeping
her mind busy and trying to understand her
perception of time. I was curious what her

responses would be. Which of her answers were consistent, which ones were true and which ones were made up? Did she even know the difference? But at the end of the day, does it really matter?

Ever since Mama was diagnosed with dementia, I was at a loss. Should I tell her? What do I say? Did the doctor tell her? How do I explain this? What is the best way to talk about it with Mama? I've always been honest with her. Questions, questions, questions.

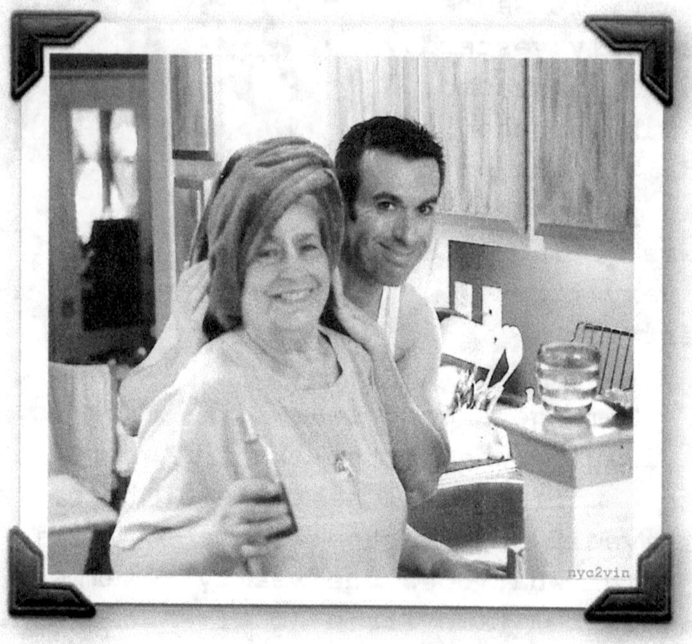

During our nightly visits it was ironic that we would help Mama try to forget. We'd pull out our bag of tricks,

put on the "happy" and distract her from
what was going on all around her. We would
try to help transport her to a better
place in time.

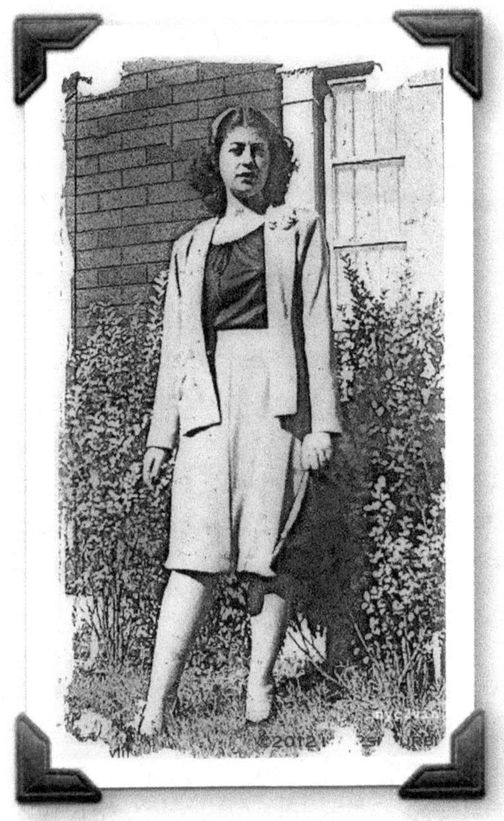

    All we really have in life is love
and memories. But sometimes it's just love
because the memories have faded. I'm lucky
enough to have both right now. Mama was
blessed to have love and lucky enough to
still be able to bullshit the rest.

My Nerves Are Shot

"My nerves are shot!" You don't know how many times I heard that from my mother, one of the original drama queens. I think the first sentence I ever formed as a child was "Mommy, mommy my nerves are shot."

My mother had me late in life, I was the miracle child. She would always talk about how long I made her suffer during labor. She carried me for nine long months and of course I was late (as usual). She endured twenty-seven excruciating hours in the delivery room and finally gave birth to me. Mama enjoyed telling this to anyone who would listen. That was the beginning of our story together and I think it explains a lot!

I'd ask her "How are you feeling tonight?" She'd say "I'm dying," then start to feign a highly dramatic cough, throw her head back and pretend that she just died. I'd say "Ma, are you okay?" She'd sit up all proper as if nothing happened. "Whaddya mean, am I okay? My nerves are shot." That was just another typical day with Mama.

Over the years, when friends would ask how we were doing, I'd say "Another

day, another dose of Mama Drama." Then it
all clicked and we crowned Anna with the
perfect title: *Dementia-Mama-Drama.*

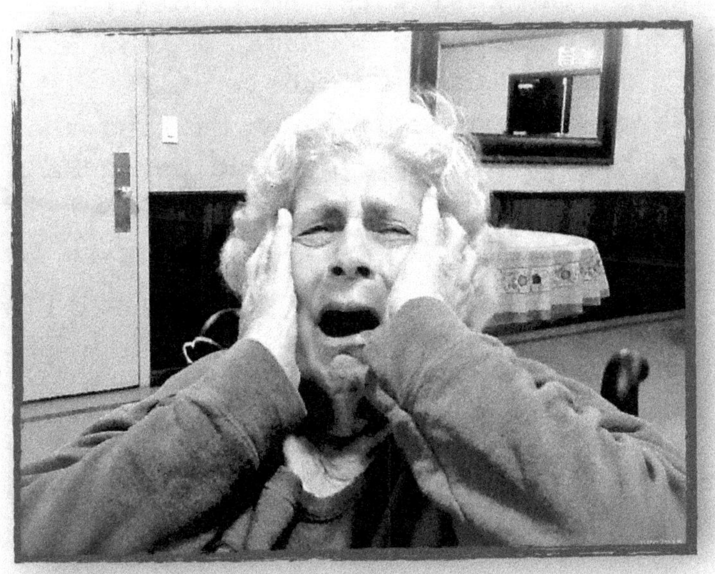

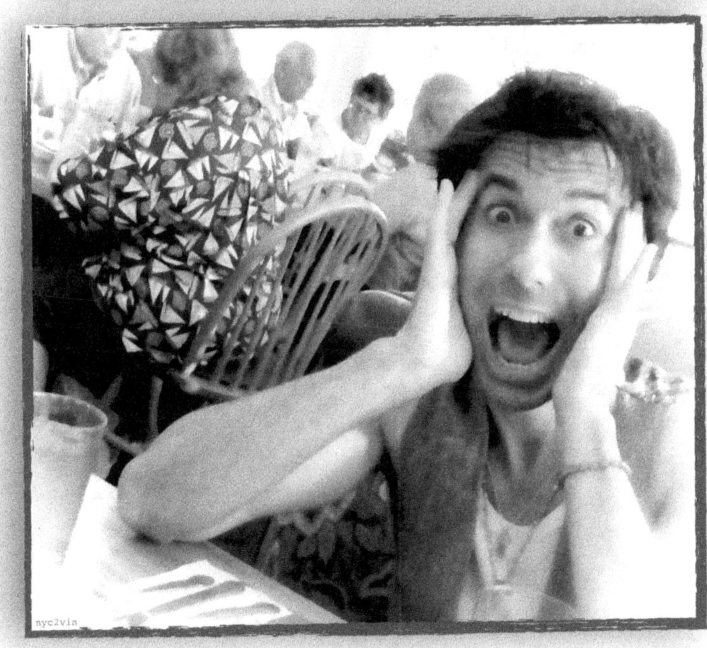

I had my own daily drama too. I had
to deal with the staff at the nursing home
- the doctors, the nurses, the social
workers, the residents, her roommate and
of course, the star... Mama. I knew every
staff members name and their shift. It was
a twenty-four hour job just getting the
phone calls from everyone including Mama.

So I told you how I came up with the
name *Dementia-Mama-Drama*, but did I tell
you that MY nerves are shot?

The Change

Even before Mama was diagnosed with dementia, the parent/child role reversal was often there. I remember when I was ten years old and Mama came home late from a doctor's appointment and I was worried...

Vin: You're late, why didn't you call? How was your appointment? What did he say?

Mama: You worry too much. He said that I'm very nervous and I need to relax.

Vin: That's what he always says. But are you okay, Ma?

Mama: Yeah, of course I'm fine. But I'm going through "the change".

Vin: What change?

Mama: "The change".

Vin: What's the change?

Mama: Your father will be home soon, ask him. Do you want some ice cream?

Years later in the nursing home, Mama's doctor visits were becoming more frequent. I didn't know exactly why, so of course I began to worry even more...

Vin: How was your doctor's visit today?
What did he say?

Mama: Ohhh, I'm just sick and tired.

Vin: He said that you're sick and tired?

Mama: No, he said I'm fine.

Vin: You're fine?

Mama: Yes, he said I'll be fine when my
son gets me the hell out of this place.

Vin: Really? That's what the doctor said?
I'll ask him about that tomorrow. Do you
want some ice cream?

Some things change and some things
don't. And so it goes...

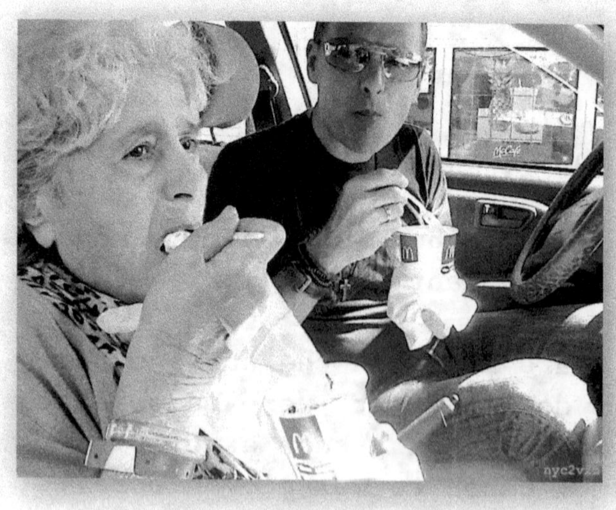

I Love You Too Dear,
But Not THAT Way

When Mama lived at The Village Nursing Home in New York, she had a lot of friends. This was a big difference from The Rafael Nursing Home in California where she had little social activity or friends. In NYC the visitors of other residents would stop by and talk to Mama and made her feel special. She looked forward to sitting outside on the bench in any weather to watch the people pass by. There was always a lot of activity and a diverse group in the Village on 12th Street. Some of them would stop and chat with her as they walked their dogs, pushed their baby strollers or on their way to or from work. Some of the people would even call her by her nickname "Anna with a Z".

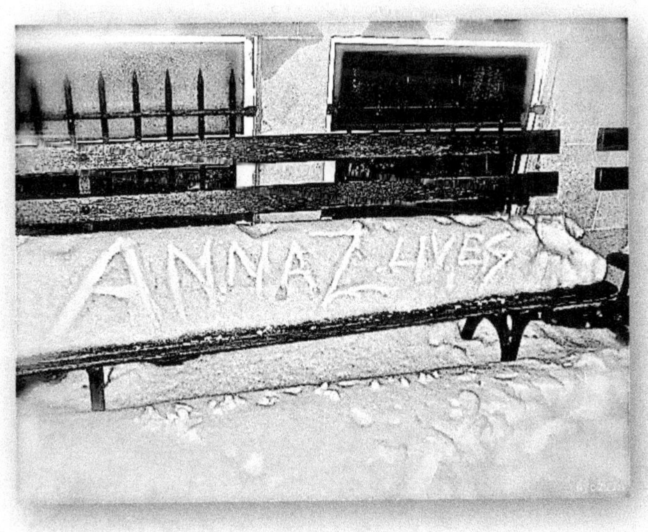

One of Mama's best friends at the Village Nursing Home was Joyce. Joyce had suffered a stroke and was wheelchair bound. She had great difficulty speaking but fortunately Mama could understand her most of the time. Joyce was a big smoker and also loved to sit outside where she could smoke. They had their spats, but through it all, they were inseparable. One of the first conversations I heard between them when I met Joyce sounded like a classic comedy routine. These two old gals *always* told it like it was...

Mama: Vincent, this is my friend Joyce.

Joyce: Hi Vincent. I'm a lesbian... well, I used to be.

Mama: That's nice dear, as long as you're happy.

Vin: Joyce, you know I'm gay too, right?

Joyce: Yeah I know. *(Pause)* Did you know my daughter is a prostitute?

Vin: No, I didn't.

Mama: Well as long as she enjoys what she's doing and she's good at it.

Vin: Ma, what are you talking about?

Joyce: Oh Vin, I LOVE your mother. *(With
some difficulty, she reached over to hold
Mama's hand.)*

Mama: *(Mama gingerly pulled her hand away
and patted Joyce on her knee)* I love you
too dear, but not THAT way.

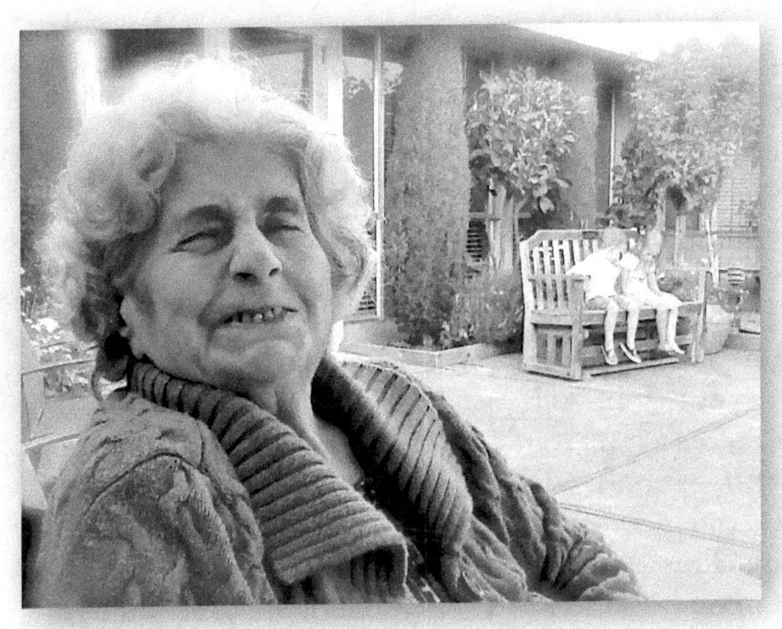

Elephants Never Forget

Elephants never forget, people do. Unfortunately like Mama, some people get Alzheimer's.

I enjoyed Yoga for many years and decided to study and get my degree so I could also teach. The concept of mind, body and spirit is very important and helpful to many. I received two degrees in Yoga, the second one being in "gentle yoga" to help Mama and others like her. When you graduate and become certified, the instructors and Swamis assign you a spiritual name. The name is carefully selected for you through their understanding of your overall persona. Most graduates will use their spiritual name when they start to teach. The name given to me was Vinayaka and I loved it.

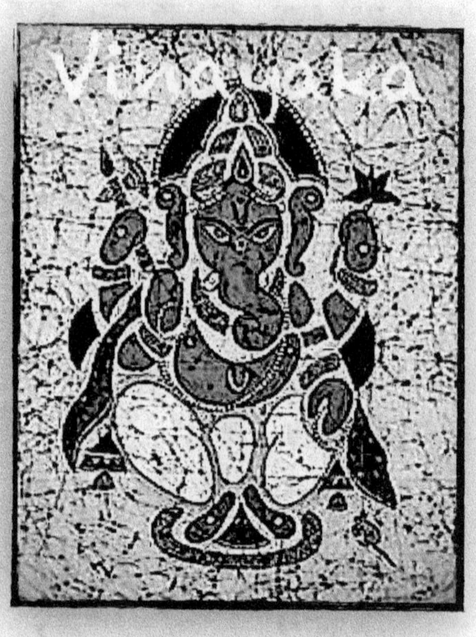

Vinayaka is a man with an elephants head and symbolizes overcoming obstacles and was the protector of his mother. How perfect, it was my life story. Overcoming obstacles was my middle name! I had a lot of obstacles every day being a caregiver for Mama. I was very attached to the name.

Vinayaka is also another name for Ganesh, a sacred deity. Many people said I was a saint when I was a caregiver, but I just did what came naturally. I learned to overcome obstacles and was the protector of Mama up until the very end. Maybe it was all something that was just meant to be. Cosmic, Karmic, call it what you want.

During our nightly routine of exercises with Mama I'd add a few Yoga exercises to the mix. It was like when a parent would sneak some vegetables into the meal. I'd add three part 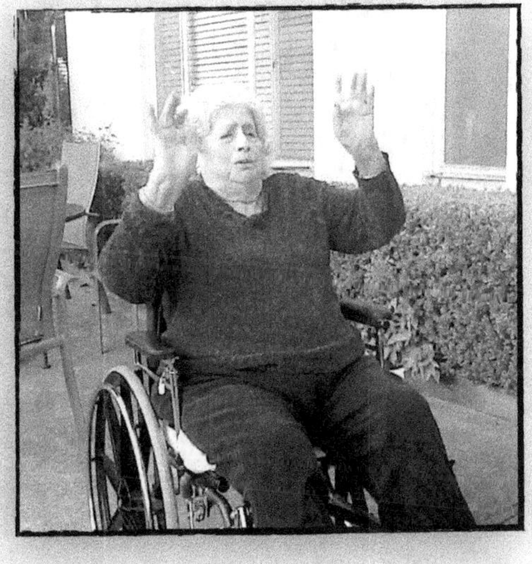 breathing, gentle basic poses and we would sometimes chant the Yogic "OM" mantra. She was a trooper and did the exercises even though she usually didn't want to do them. Mama always got a kick out of the chanting

because she loved to sing. She preferred
show tunes, but who wouldn't? She didn't
know what she was chanting and it always
made her laugh. She'd say "If anybody
heard me, they'd think I was crazy." Her
laugh was contagious and the three of us
couldn't stop laughing.

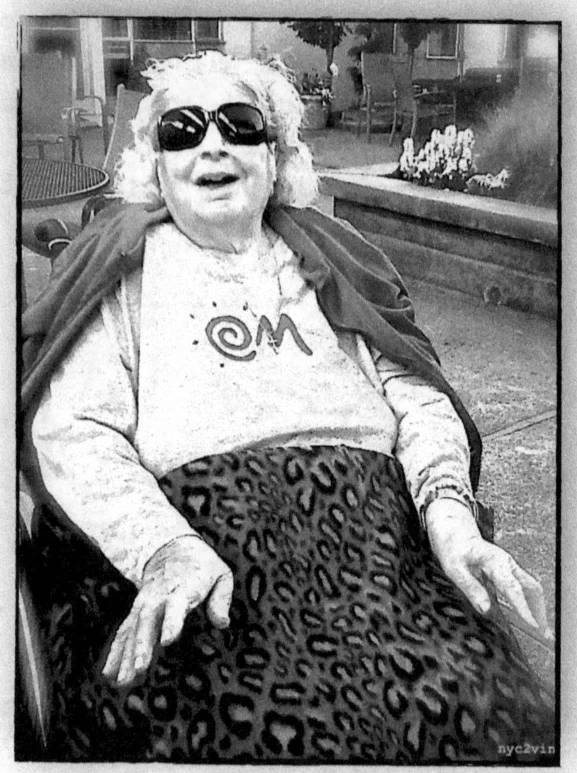

    Laughter is one of the things that
always helped us overcome our obstacles
and that's what this "elephant" will never
forget.

Gotta Sing For My Supper

The days were long for both of us for different reasons. Hers was because of her dementia, confusion and loneliness. Mine was because of the constant challenge of being a caregiver while trying to balance our everyday life and keeping any plans tentative. This day was not a good one for me and I guess it was obvious.

Mama was sitting in the empty dining room at a table watching the large screen tv. She had a napkin on her blouse as if she was waiting for dinner to be served, but it had many food stains on it so I knew she had already eaten. It was well after dinner time and all the tables had been cleared.

Mama: What's the matter?

Vin: I don't feel so great.

Mama: So what are you doing here? Whaddya want? If ya want sympathy go to the card store, haha!

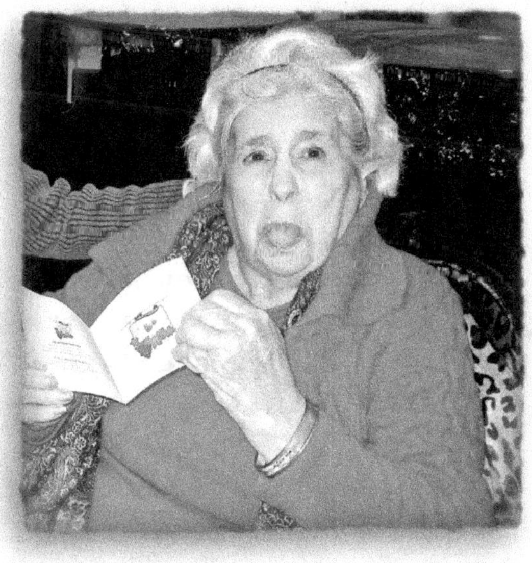

Vin: Is that any way to talk to your son?

Mama: Gimme a break will ya. What about the way you talked to me when you were a teenager?

Vin: What are you talking about? You can't remember what you had for dinner but you can remember that?

Mama: Dinner? I'm still waiting for my dinner.

Vin: Ma you're full of shit, you ate dinner over two hours ago.

Mama: Oh, go to hell, why don't ya. I'm starving, starving! You always had a potty mouth.

Vin: A potty mouth? Who do you think I got it from?

Mama: How would I know? All I know is I want my dinner.

Vin: I can't follow this conversation anymore. I'll just ask the nurse to bring you some coffee and cake. In the meantime, why don't you sing me a song?

Mama: Sing? You want me to sing a song now too? What do I gotta sing for my supper?

Vin: **Ma, you love to sing.**

Mama: **Yeah I love to sing but I also love
to eat and I didn't eat yet!**

Vin: **Well sing me a song for now.**

Mama: **Jesus Christ, you want all of me?**

Vin: **What?**

Mama: **Do you want me to sing "All of Me"?**

Vin: **Yeah sing it and swing it.**

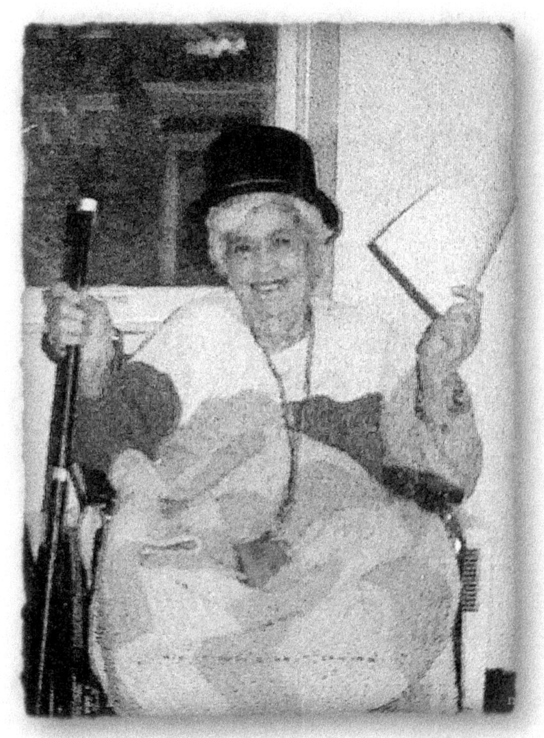

    She sang a swingy version of the
song several times as some of the staff
applauded her as they passed by the dining
room. Her coffee and cake arrived and she
stopped singing.

Vin: I needed that song. It's just what
the doctor ordered, I feel better now.

Mama: Good, now can I have my dinner?

Vin: We've been through this, you already
had your dinner. Now enjoy your cake and
coffee.

Mama: Oh Jesus, you have no sympathy.

Vin: Sympathy? Like you said before, if ya
want sympathy go to the card store, haha!
Goodnight Ma.

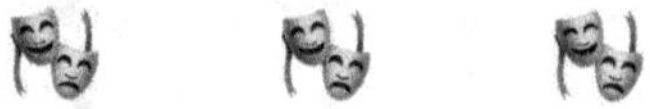

I'm NOT A Saint

When I became a caregiver for Mama people would always tell me that I was a saint. I gotta be totally honest, I am NOT a saint, not even close to one. On the other hand, Douglass *was* a saint. He put up with Mama AND me! Douglass knew my mom before dementia. Once she was diagnosed and I took my role as caregiver, I thought this could be the end of our relationship. Luckily he stepped up and was the calming supportive caregiver that I needed too.

We worked well together, he'd calm Mama down as I took care of dealing with the nurses and staff, he even did her nails! We were fortunate that it brought us closer together. I tend to overreact *(wonder where that comes from)* and he was much more patient.

There are many levels and emotions to being a caregiver, it's hard to explain. The best analogy for me would be like having a child when you never planned on one, but wouldn't change it if you could.

There were days I had to distance myself and think of myself first. They were rare, but I did have them. Those were the days when the Italian Catholic guilt entered the picture. I felt like our lives were constantly on hold. Sometimes I just wanted to run away from the entire role of caregiver and leave it all for someone else. The problem was there really wasn't anyone else. Besides I would NEVER do that to my mother.

There were other days that would remind me of when I was growing up and how Mama and I would constantly challenge each other. The roles may have changed, but the dynamics and the show were still the same.

Thankfully, there were days when I could enjoy it all for what it was and be grateful that I still had Mama. We laughed, sang, reminisced, made up stories and played cards. Those are the parts I prefer to remember and to let you know

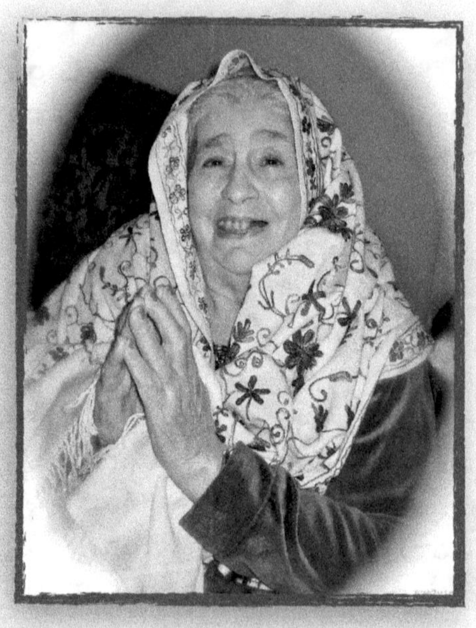

there can *still* be good days... if you just "let go" and try to be in the moment.

Being a caregiver and always trying to "fix it" wore me out. I didn't realize

it at the time, I just did what I needed
to do. I'd always be on call leaving my
phone on 24/7. I did this for thirteen
years and didn't realize what a physical
as well as emotional toll it took on me.
Then one day the phone stopped ringing. A
relief? Yes, but no.

    One of Mama's favorite saints was
Saint Jude which is the saint of lost
causes. It's ironic that Alzheimer's
Disease has been considered a lost cause
to some, but to me it was just another
part of our lives and another challenge.
Mama's other favorite saint *(she had many)*
was Saint Theresa - "little flower show
your power in my most needed hour." I'm
not a saint, but perhaps being there in
her most needed hour made me a saint to
her, *just don't call me Theresa!*

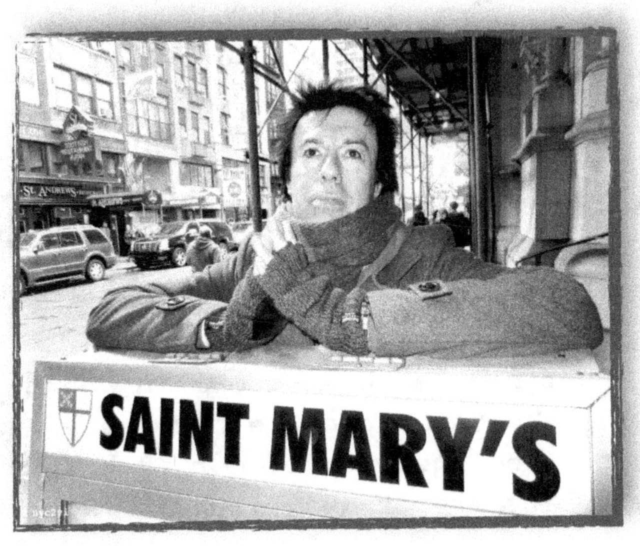

Dealing With Mama

   Mama loved playing cards. It was a
good distraction and a familiar routine
for her. We always played her version of
gin rummy. It became our ritual and we
could tell if it was a good night or not
depending on how long she wanted to play.
It was our comfort zone. No more questions
and no more complaining... we were all in
the moment. It took our minds off of what
was going on *and* it was fun. It made her
think and made us all laugh.

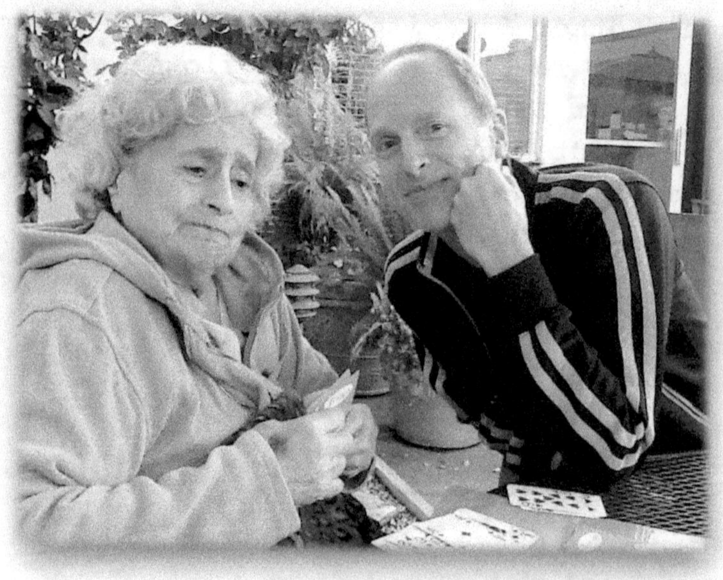

   Most nights she'd complain about
dealing the cards because her hands hurt
so much from the pain of her arthritis. I
didn't let her get away with it, Douglass

on the other hand was more forgiving. We
both knew it was good exercise for her
arthritic hands and could help with her
concentration, so I insisted she had to
deal. Mama was a very serious card player
and sometimes she could add up the final
scores quicker than Douglass or I.

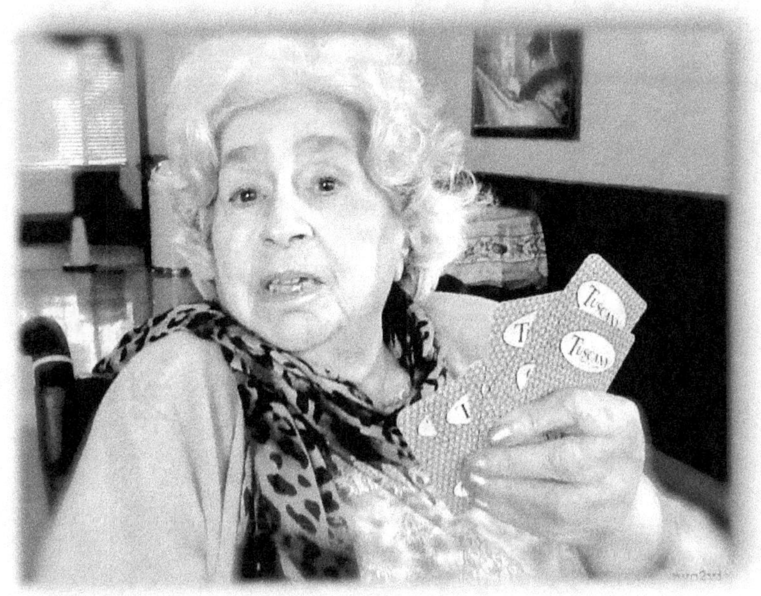

Playing cards was also a part of her
past. She always loved playing cards with
my father, her friends or the family. It
wasn't only the weekly late night card
games they had but also the games they had
after family gatherings. Mama was the
"hostess with the mostest" as she sweetly
brought out snacks but then cursed when
she was losing! My father would just shake
his head and laugh.

We'd play cards with Mama until she got tired or couldn't concentrate any longer. We were always dealing with Mama as caregivers daily *but* when it came to our nightly card games, we just played cards... *dealing with Mama.*

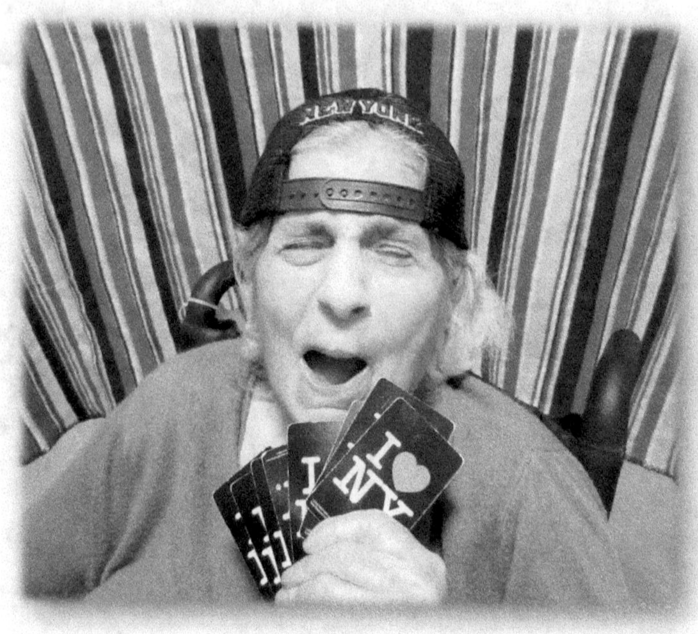

Money? I Have Some Money

During a visit with Mama one night we were cleaning out her purse. We did this often because she would wrap and save food she didn't finish at mealtime to keep for later. Her purse was always full of stuff, we even found her tv remote in there. She tried to help by pulling out her leopard coin purse. She took out a dollar bill, looked at it and then put it back in. She did this repeatedly as we continued to clean out her purse. So then we started to talk about money...

Vin: Why haven't you ever saved any money?

Mama: Vincent your father was a gambler, that son of a bitch, may he rest in peace.

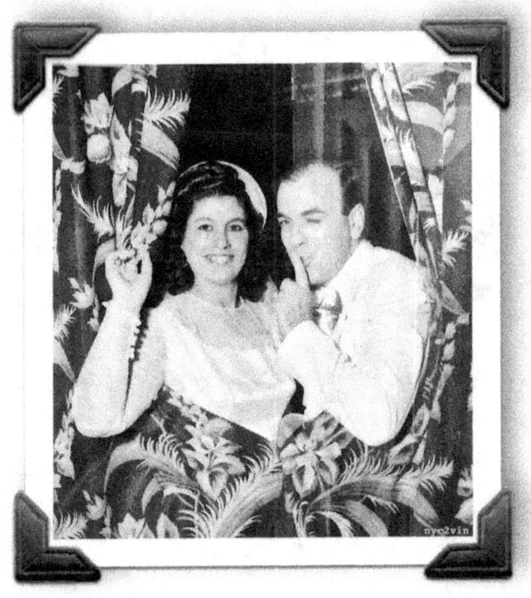

He ran the numbers, he was a bookie. Don't you remember taking the numbers on the phone for him on Saturday mornings? He slept late after playing cards all night and I wouldn't take the numbers. We never could save a damn dime!

Vin: Well, why didn't you try to save some money on your own?

Mama: Money? I have some money.

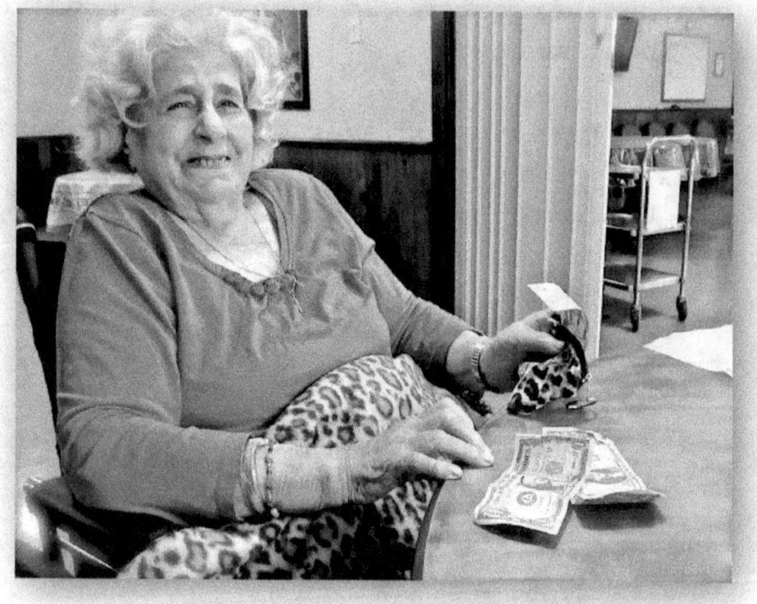

Vin: You do?

Mama: Sure, I have a couple of hundred in my bank account. When I drop dead, you'll have a couple of hundred.

Douglass and I started laughing which
made Mama start laughing. We knew she
didn't have a bank account for many years.
I gave her two more dollars to put in her
coin purse.

Mama: What's this for?

Vin: That's for making us laugh.

Mama: *(She looked at us and gave a big
smile)* I should make you laugh more often.

It was a good night, and definitely
worth the two bucks!

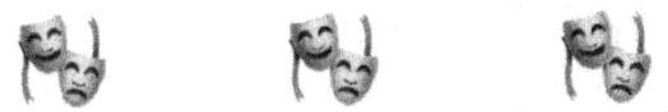

Mama Was Everyone's Mother

I remember when I was growing up, Mama was a mother to everyone. Not only to the family but to my friends and even the neighborhood kids. They all loved her and she loved them. She had thirteen brothers and sisters growing up and lost her mother at a very young age, so she was a natural caregiver. Everyone knew "Anna with a Z". She was the one you could talk to about anything. They always wanted to hang out at our apartment. It may have been small but it was the place to be. She was a great cook and there was always lots of food ready to be put on the table.

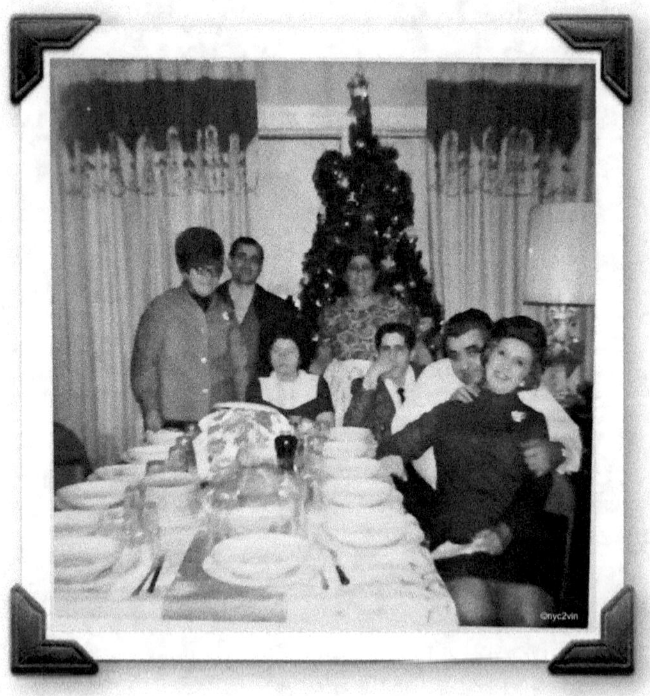

Time moves on and things change. The
tables have turned and no one was sitting
at her table any longer. She was still
Anna, but was she? She often felt lonely,
isolated and even forgotten.

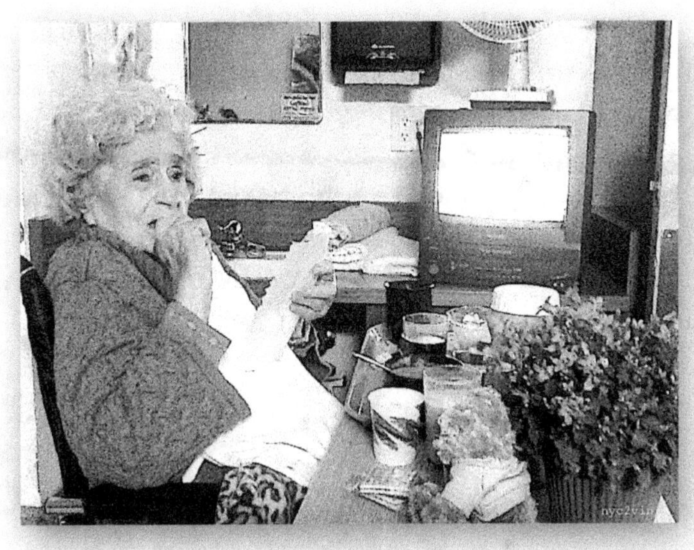

It was Mother's Day and she asked me
repeatedly, "Where is everybody?" I tried
to smooth it over and explain that people
have their own lives and most don't live
nearby anymore. One minute she'd say "The
hell with them" and the next minute she
would revel in her glory days remembering
her "children" - nieces, nephews and my
friends. She told stories about taking
some of them to Radio City Music Hall,
seeing Sinatra at The Paramount, visiting
The Botanical Gardens or The Bronx Zoo.
These were feel good memories for Mama.

I stopped trying to make excuses for
what wasn't and tried to focus on what
was... just being in the moment with Mama.
I was always aware that it could be the
last Mother's Day that she'd remember.

We made an extra effort to be sure
that she wasn't in the nursing home
especially on Mother's Day. We would
always take her out to a restaurant to be
surrounded by people who were celebrating.
I just wanted her to feel like she was
sitting at a full table once again and not
alone.

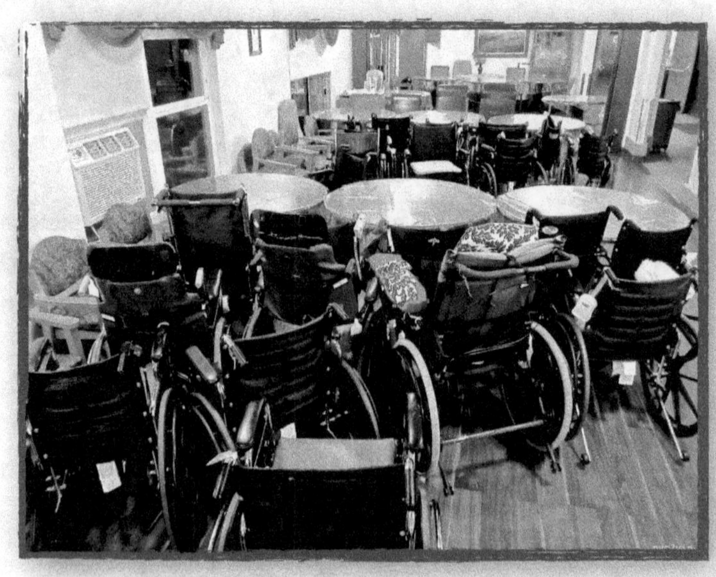

Movin' With Mama

Mama didn't move many times in her life. She grew up in Harlem and my parents lived in the same apartment in the Bronx for almost forty years, all she knew was New York. Her first big move came when she wasn't able to take care of herself and live alone any longer. She needed to be in

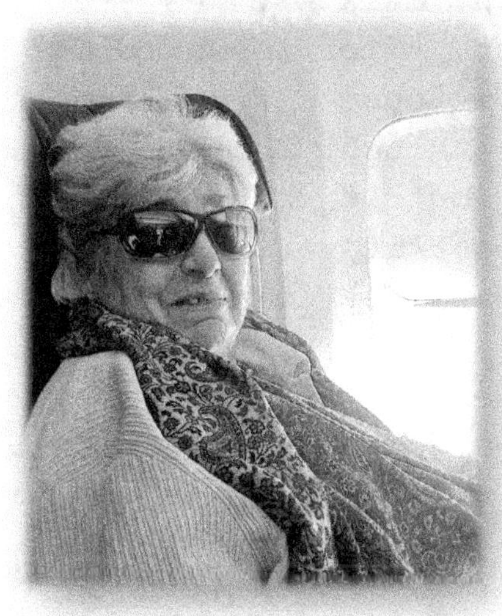

a nursing home. It was very important she was nearby. I really pushed to get her into The Village Nursing Home just a block away from Douglass and me. It was almost as tough as getting your child into a good school!

After she lived there for nine years the nursing home was sold and would be closing. We were very anxious and didn't know what to do. I looked for places to move Mama, but there weren't any nearby. As this drama was going on, Douglass' mother in California became very sick. We received a phone call that she was getting worse and immediately flew to see her. When we got there she was too weak to do anything that we had hoped

to do with her. Just a few days later, she
passed away.

After returning home to New York we
had timely decisions to make. There now
was an opportunity to move to California
where it would be more affordable and a
much needed change from the city. Fast
forward, Douglass and I moved into his
mom's place and brought Mama with us, it
all happened very fast. After researching
many nursing homes, we found a few nearby.
We picked one that we thought would be a
great place for Mama, but it wasn't all it
appeared to be. At least it was within
walking distance from us and it had a
beautiful garden.

We packed up Mama for her very first
plane ride.
Knowing her
anxieties, I
worried that she
might freak out
but she loved
it! She sang
"California Here
I Come" in the
cab ride to the
airport, on the
plane *(many
times)* and when
we landed.

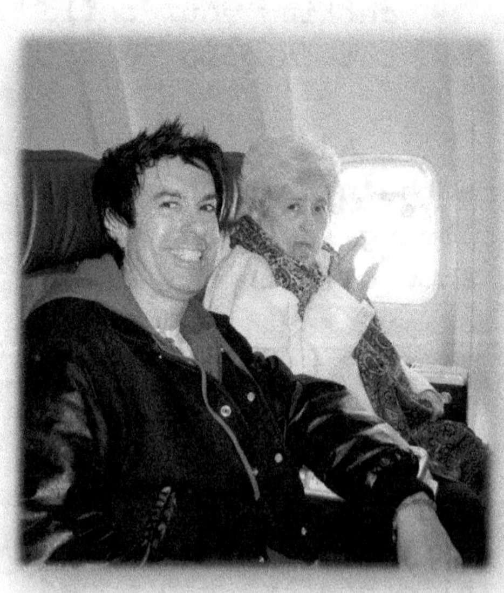

Her first flight had to be special so
we flew first class. Our plan was to keep
her distracted. We kept her entertained
the entire flight by singing and watching
video clips of old musical numbers and
playing tic-tac-toe. When this didn't work
we'd plug her into our iPod. The earbuds
kept falling out and she'd curse out loud,
it was quite comical. She kept saying that
she loved the flight and felt like the
plane was hardly moving. Thank God, the
flight was a hit. She was in seventh
heaven eating nonstop and lucky for us
they served lasagna. The biggest treat for
Mama was when they rolled the ice cream
cart down the aisle and she had a custom
made sundae with the works.

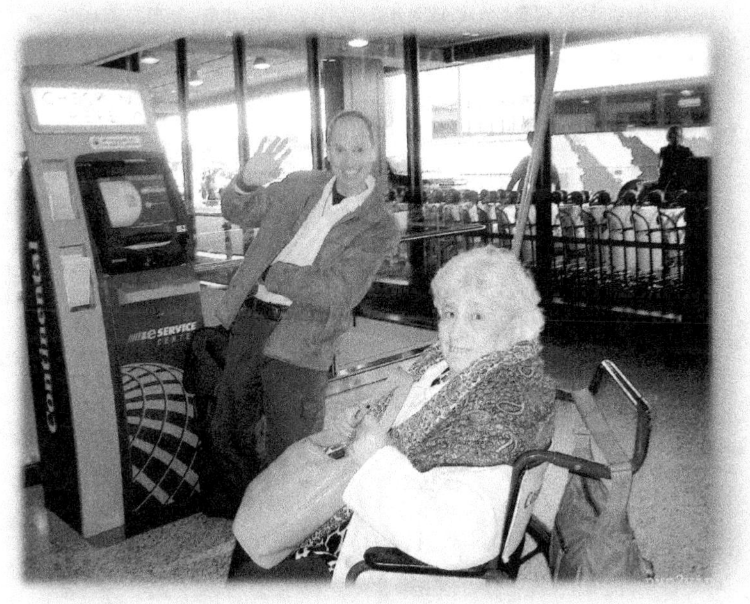

When we landed we were exhausted but still had to drive from the airport to the new nursing home. For Mama the reality of being in a different place, in a different bed and in a different time zone was overwhelming. Everything must have set in and she had a meltdown. She was crying hysterically and not making much sense. She didn't even care about the beautiful rainbow that appeared as we drove over the Golden Gate Bridge. Douglass and I looked at each other and started to doubt our decision to move.

After checking into the nursing home and putting her into bed, we stayed with her until she was finally calm and fell asleep. When Douglass and I got to our new place we ordered takeout, then we just collapsed and went to bed. For better or worse we were ready to begin our new chapter in suburbia.

Yes Sir, That's My Baby

As I walked into Mama's room, I noticed she had her eyes closed and was humming. She was clutching one of her stuffed animals. She won them as prizes at the nursing home during bingo games. Mama always loved bingo as far back as I could remember. She would go to bingo halls or the church with my father to play. After he died, she'd go with her friends to play. We even played after family dinners as a child, because who doesn't have a bingo game at home? After bingo the cards came out for the adults.

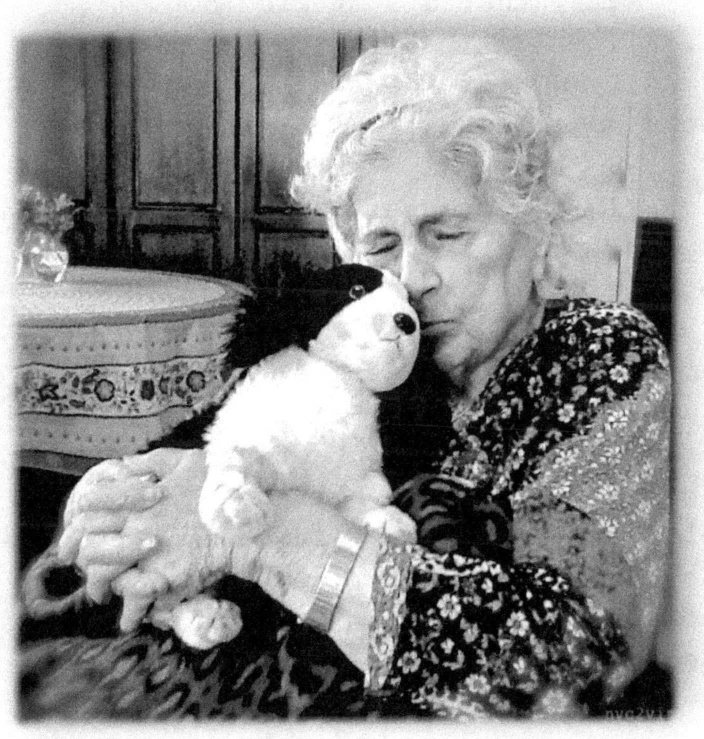

This night she seemed like she was in another world with her stuffed dog. Was she thinking it was one of her dogs from her past? She looked up at me and caught me off guard...

Vin: **Mama, what the hell are you doing?**

Mama: **I'm singing to my baby.**

Vin: *(I started to freak out a little)* **What do you mean your baby?**

Mama: **That's my baby.**

Vin: **Mama, that's a stuffed dog.**

Mama: **I KNOW it's a stuffed dog, but it keeps me company.**

Vin: *(Thank God she knew it was a stuffed dog and not a baby)* **Glad you have company. So what song were you humming?**

Mama: **"Yes sir, that's my baby."**

I wheeled her out of her room as she continued to cuddle her dog. I knew she felt helpless because she couldn't operate the wheelchair on her own, even after repeated lessons. In New York she always used her walker but was now confined to a wheelchair after moving to California.

The transition was very upsetting for Mama because she lost another level of her independence. I fought and fought but they never allowed her to use her walker again. It was a losing battle.

I wheeled her into the garden for a change of scenery. It was a beautiful warm summer night and we both started to sing the song together.

"Yes sir, that's my baby. No sir, I don't mean maybe. Yes sir, that's my baby now..."

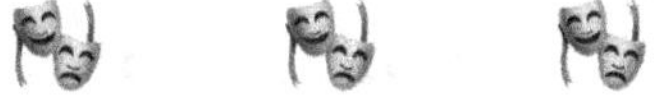

Any Phone Calls Today?

We noticed Mama was a little sad when we got to her room, so we wheeled her out to the garden which usually helped her mood. It was a very lush colorful garden with purple bougainvilleas, many fragrant roses and a tranquil fountain. We tried to see where the sadness was coming from...

Douglass: You don't seem too happy. What's going on with you today Anna?

Mama: Ohhh, ya don't wanna know. When I look in the mirror I say what the hell! Who is *that* woman? That's not me, that's some other me.

Vin: No Ma, that's you, you're old. We're all getting old.

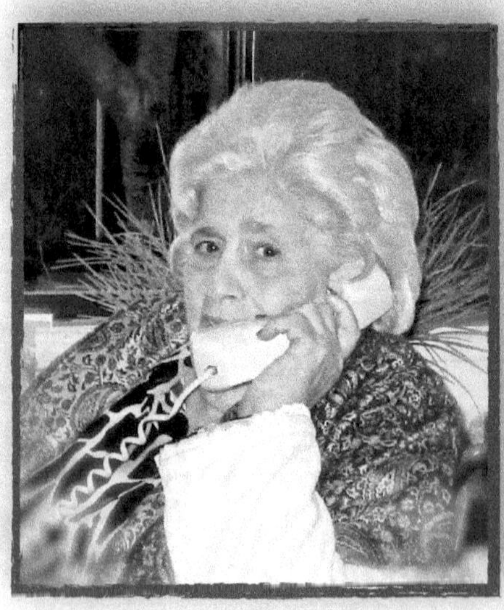

Mama: But nobody sees me, I don't even see me. Everybody has forgotten me. I've even forgotten me.

Vin: Come on, nobody has forgotten you.

Douglass: Any
phone calls
today?

Mama: Nah,
they're all
dead. Dead!

Douglass: Who
is all dead?
What are you
talking about
Anna?

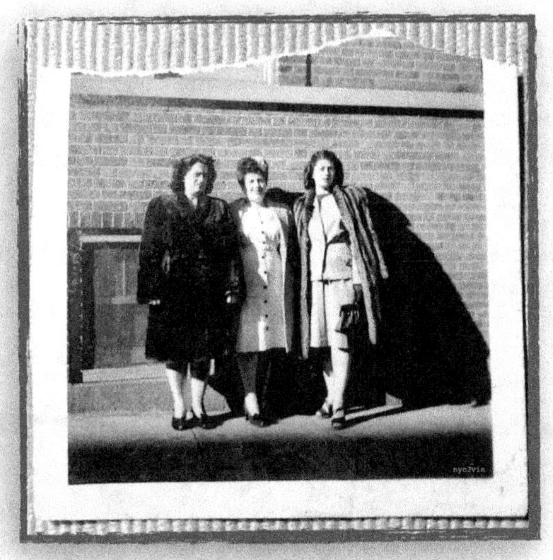

Mama: They're ALL dead to me. My family!
They can't even call me.

Vin: Okay, so you didn't get any phone
calls today. Maybe someone will call you
tomorrow.

Mama: Nah, no one is gonna call me. I
dream of my mother and she doesn't call
me. Not even my sisters or your Aunt Jo,
she didn't call me today.

Vin: But Ma, you know Aunt Jo has been
dead for years.

Mama: Ohhh my God! What the hell am I
talking about? I'm waiting for a phone
call from a dead woman. Guess it'll be one
hell of a long wait.

Day Care Dilemma

I finally knew what it must have felt like for Mama to let go of her fat little crying boy and send him to kindergarten. I had the same anxious feeling when I sent Mama to senior day care.

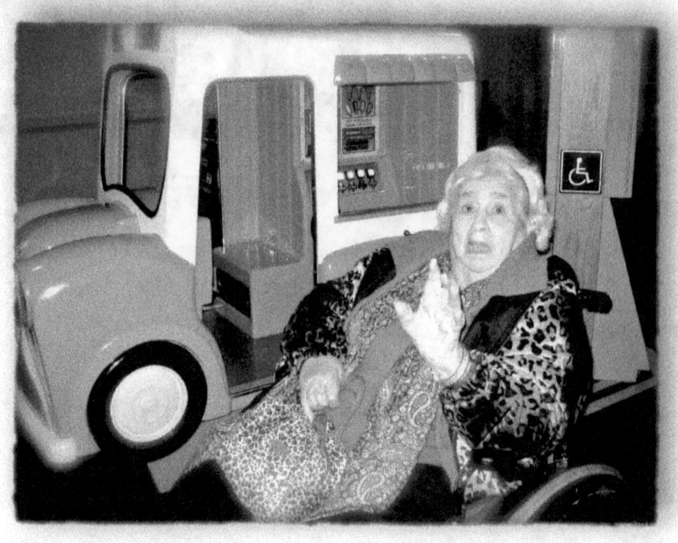

I thought it would have been a good change for Mama to get out of the nursing home a few times a week. She'd have a scenic ride in a van, be in a different environment or make new friends *and* engage in activities. These were things that she missed and would complain about not having at the nursing home. I thought the perfect solution would be senior day care. On her first day, of course she took center stage and sang a song, just like I did on my first day of kindergarten when I sang

"Somewhere Over The Rainbow." But that didn't last long, she gradually turned into the child I was in kindergarten. She would often get combative, refusing to go back to "school". The nursing home called me often to help coax her into going while the van was waiting. This perfect solution was not working out *and* it was expensive.

I tried reasoning with her repeatedly but as time went by I realized the bottom line was that Mama needed her routine. She didn't like change even though the nursing home was less than perfect. She complained that "There's no life here and there's nothing to do in this damn joint." It was easier for her to stay there and complain, it was her comfort zone.

After a few months, I gave in to Mama just like she always gave into me as a child. I told her that she didn't have to go to day care anymore if she didn't want to go. She was relieved and seemed just as happy 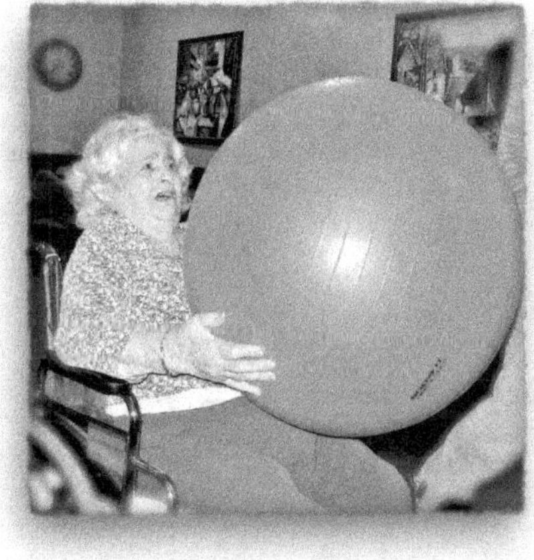 as I did when she told me I could miss school. We spoiled each other. We were two of a kind and it came around full circle.

Ya Gotta Have A Big Mouth

Once again it pays to have a big mouth and ask a lot of questions. It was Mama's fourth ER visit within the last six months for another blood transfusion. If I didn't push for her to be released from the hospital, she would have been there all weekend. Usually not much gets done in hospitals on the weekends.

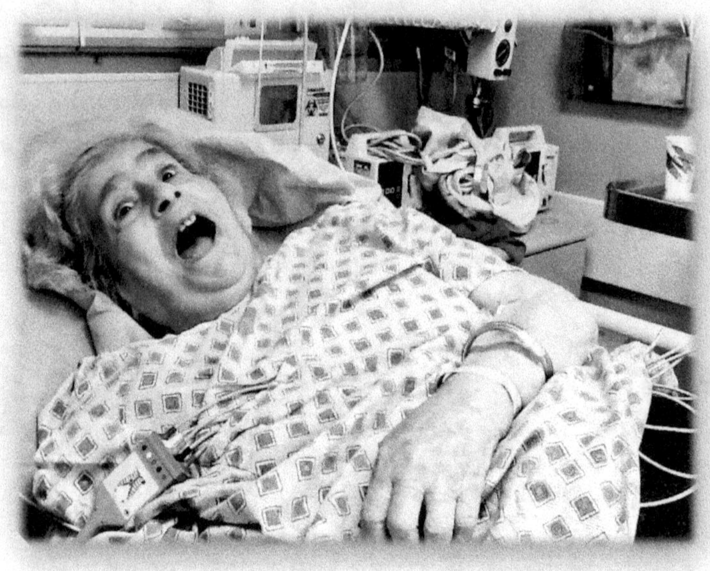

Vin: *(Talking to the head nurse)* Are you sure we need *another* test? The last test wasn't even necessary, I want to speak to the doctor. Mama received her transfusion overnight and it's been finished for hours. She's very anxious about getting back to the nursing home and I want her to

be released. She doesn't need to get more
agitated and disoriented. You do remember
that she has dementia?

Nurse: Oh that's right she has dementia, I
forgot. Well, the doctor won't be here for
a few more hours.

Vin: Oh, really? I just heard the doctor
being paged. I need to speak to the doctor
and clarify the situation NOW. All I need
is a minute of her time.

After more persuasion and refusing to
take NO for an answer the doctor magically
appeared within minutes. She agreed with
me that Mama
didn't need
any further
tests and
could leave.
So I was right
again and
another test
was not
needed. She
would have
stayed in the
hospital the
entire weekend
for another
unnecessary
test. WTF?

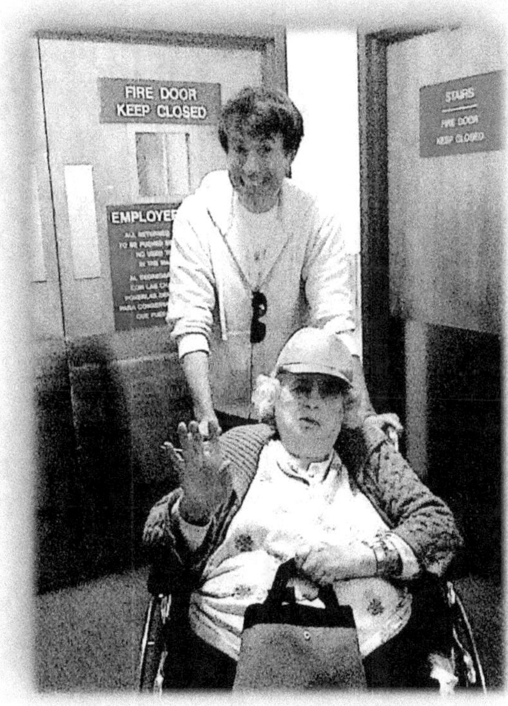

It would have caused Mama even more
anxiety and more confusion staying in an
unfamiliar place. We packed her up and got
her out of there immediately... *Phewww!*

My advice for other caregivers is to
speak up, don't take NO for an answer and
keep asking questions, REPEAT yourself.
Keep repeating to everyone: the nurses,
the doctors and the staff. YOU know your
loved one more than anyone in the ER does,
especially a doctor seeing them for the
first time. Keep the information of your
loved one easily accessible in your phone.
Their medical history, medication list,
any notes or questions, etc.

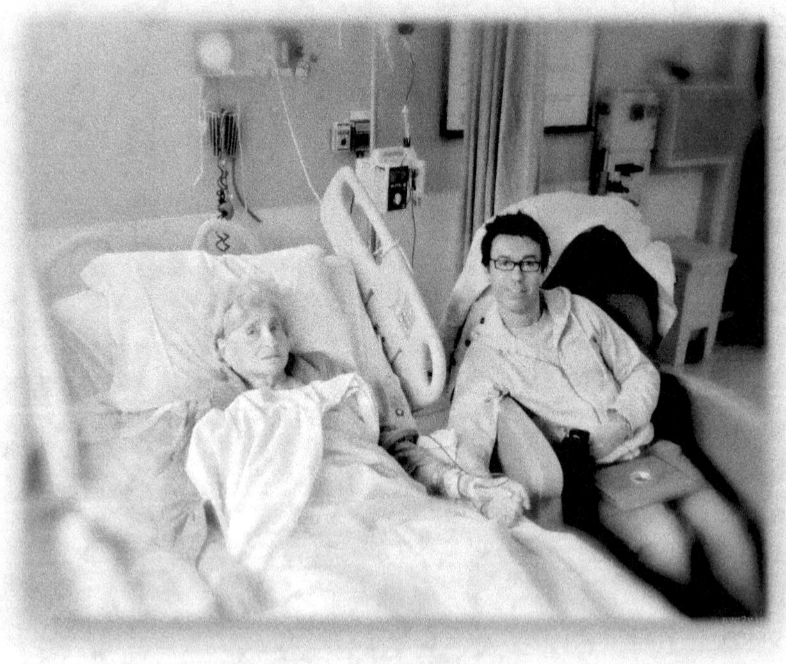

From my experience, most nurses and
doctors do not always fully read the
charts. Shifts change and they probably
will ask the same questions, when the
answers are already noted in the charts.
Be the squeaky wheel, don't be afraid to
speak up. Question everything and always
ask about *any* alternative options. Don't
just accept the first suggestion given.
Tell them what you feel your loved one
needs. Think Shirley MacLaine in "Terms of
Endearment" - *"Give my daughter the shot
NOW... Thank you..."*

At times it may seem like an uphill
battle but it's just another challenge to
overcome. Hang in there, you know you can
do it, ya just gotta have a big mouth!

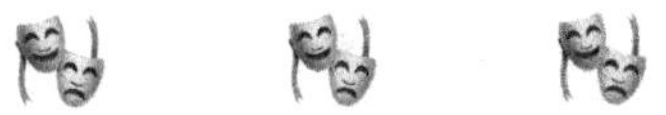

In A Mood

It was constantly an emotional roller coaster with Mama Drama, as cliché as it may sound. From the moment I entered her room I could usually tell by her face, how she was doing and what kind of mood I'd have to deal with that day.

I was not in the best of moods after an exhausting day as I got to her room. When I said hello, she barely had any energy and hardly a light of recognition upon seeing me. She was in an odd mood. Normally she'd be happy I was there or start complaining about something and *always* ask for food. I knew it would be a challenging visit.

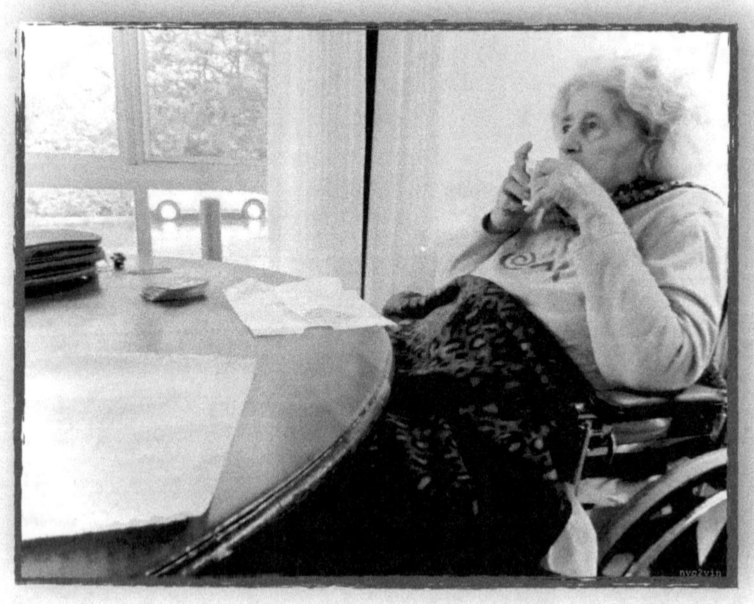

Vin: Do you want some chocolate?

Mama: Whaddya think? *(She took it and finally a little smile appeared)*

Vin: Do you want to get out of your room and play some cards?

Mama: Of course! Let's play some cards already. My hands are killing me, so you gotta deal.

Okay, we were batting a thousand so far, thank God. I just didn't have the energy to put on a show and work so hard that night. Like most caregivers, there were other things I had to deal with in my life besides Mama. I just wanted to stay home and relax for a change but there wasn't anyone else that visits. I slowly wheeled her out of her room and she mumbled something.

Vin: What? I can't hear you.

Mama: I said I LOVE you.

Oh my God, instead of being in the moment, I was somewhere else. This was what was important, *this* very special moment.

Vin: I love you too Mama.

Mama: I don't know what I'd do without
you.

Vin: Well, don't worry, I'll always be
here.

At times I was overwhelmed, feeling
like I was the only one who could make her
smile or change her mood. Some days I was
angry, but couldn't show it. Other days
I'd just break down in the car after I
left. Obviously, some days were more
difficult than others. I knew it was okay
to ask for help but I didn't always do it.
I learned the hard way that sometimes a
caregiver needs a caregiver too.

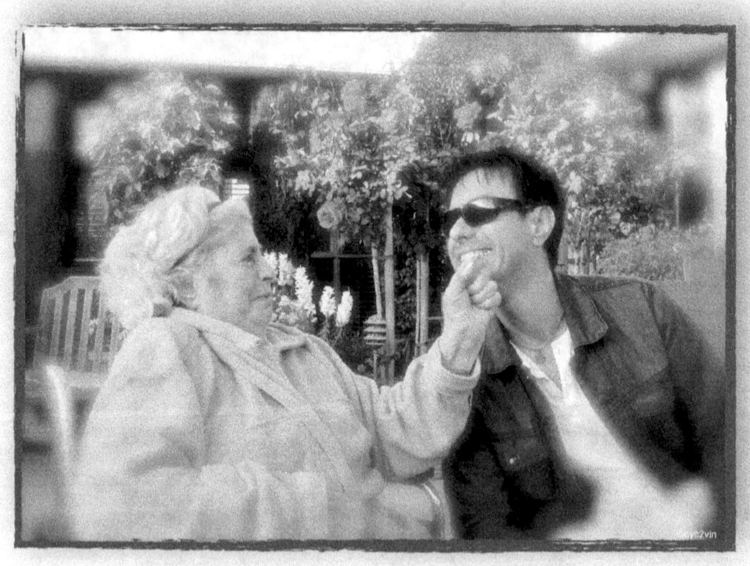

Thankfully her mood changed that
night and she started singing an uptempo

version of "Baby Face" replacing many of
the original words.

I knew that she was singing about me
because of the way she looked at me. She
sang with such devotion and motherly love
that it made everything else seem less
important. I just wanted to forget about
the day and enjoy Mama's version of the
song. It made me smile and forget my
troubles seeing the spark of energy that
was missing from her earlier that night. I
applauded her when she finished and I
thanked her with a silly grin on my face.
She said "You're welcome, son."

I left the nursing home in a good
mood and knew she was in a good mood too.
Mama was ready for bed and I was ready to
go home to relax with dinner and wine.

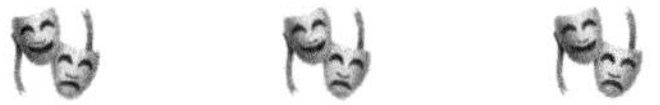

Magic Of Music

If all we really have are memories,
what happens when you no longer have any
memories? Do you have nothing? No sense or
recollection of yourself as a person? If
music can spark a memory and make you have
a sense of life and who you are, then
isn't music one of the most essential
elements in the memory making process?
Music *is* memories. Music makes you feel,
it creates an energy, it sparks life and
rhythm. I know this, I lived this.

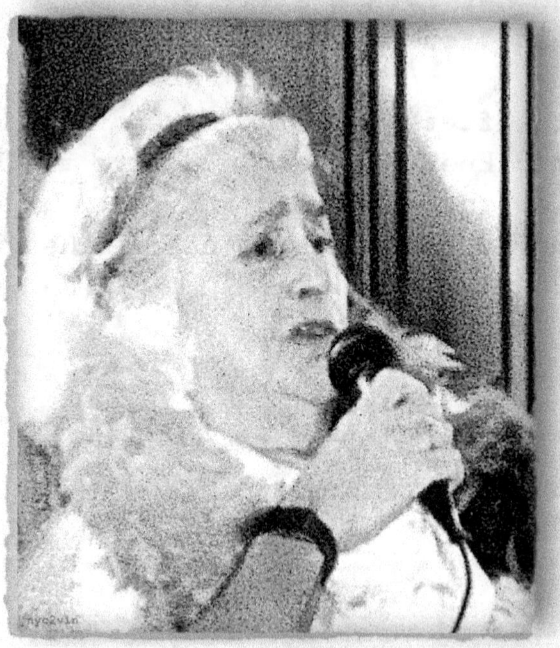

I've seen, heard and felt the magic
of music and what it did for Mama. One
late afternoon I remember entering Mama's

room and she was in her own little world
singing very softly. It was very unlike
Mama, she usually sang loudly.

Vin: Is something the matter?

Mama: I feel blue today.

Vin: Well you don't sound blue, you were
singing beautifully.

Mama: Thank you, but I sing so I don't
feel blue.

Vin: Well that's good, then you keep on
singing because you don't look blue
either. You look pretty all dressed up in
purple.

She looked at her blouse and scarf
realizing she was wearing purple and
laughed. Without missing a beat, she
smiled, looked out the window, and sang
"Blue Skies" loudly.

Music worked for Mama. She became
alive with music and magically her essence
was revitalized. She remembered words to
songs that I couldn't remember even if I
tried. We would always sing at the oddest
times... during blood transfusions, in the
ambulance and during her first (and only)
plane ride.

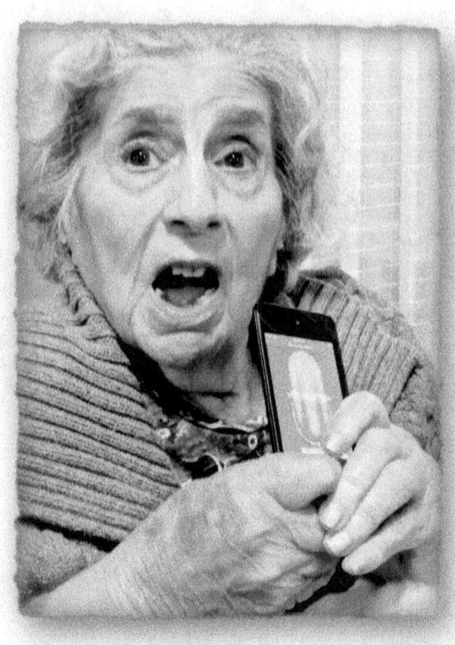

When Mama left this world Douglass and I had her favorite music playing, it was Judy Garland. I sang along as I held her hand. Music was her comfort zone and when she sang everyone around her felt good or at least smiled. We made sure that Mama was in her comfort zone when she left us and of course it was on a high note from Judy.

Music has the power to help you forget and the magic to help you remember. There's nothing else like it.

Singing The Transfusion Confusion Blues

It was Sunday and once again we were in the hospital, Mama was getting *another* blood transfusion. We would call these days our "Transfusion Confusion Daze" because we still didn't know why Mama needed those transfusions so often. No one had the answer yet. We found out much later that it was myelodysplasia (MDS) a form of leukemia. As usual Mama got confused from

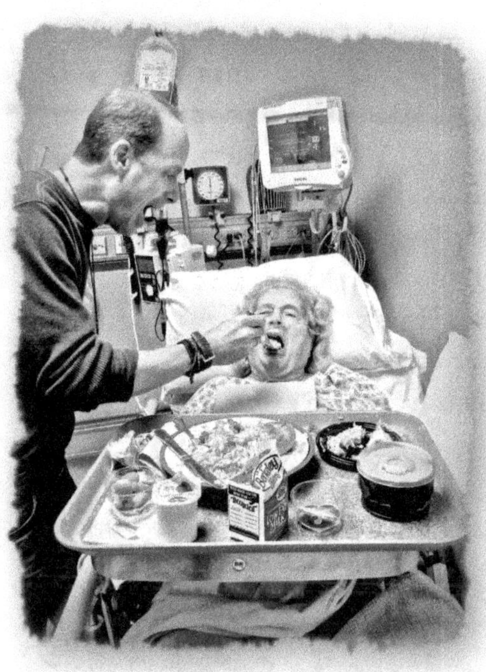

being in a new environment. It was going to be another long overnight procedure. In between complaining, napping, talking and eating, she started singing. And once she started singing, she wouldn't stop because singing was always a part of her life.

As far back as I can remember, Mama's brothers and sisters sang and played their

guitars at family gatherings. There was
constantly music in the house. When I
asked her about those times she'd say
"When my brothers sang and played, I felt
like a kid again. Ohhh, how I miss those
times. We had a ball singing together."

She would tell me stories of how she
always wanted to be a singer when she was
growing up. As a child, she often sang on
a kiddie radio shows. I remember the sound
and the joy in her voice singing in
church. So it's not a surprise that she
was transformed when she sang. Songs
triggered memories, even those we thought
she lost. Her memories were still attached
to the songs she sang. Music helped make

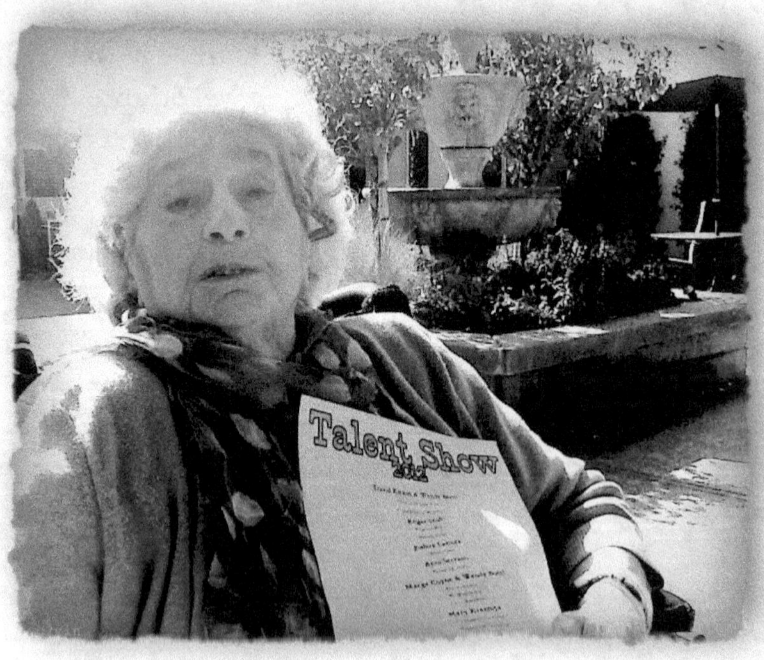

her happy and kept her alive during her last years. She loved to hear the sound of her own voice!

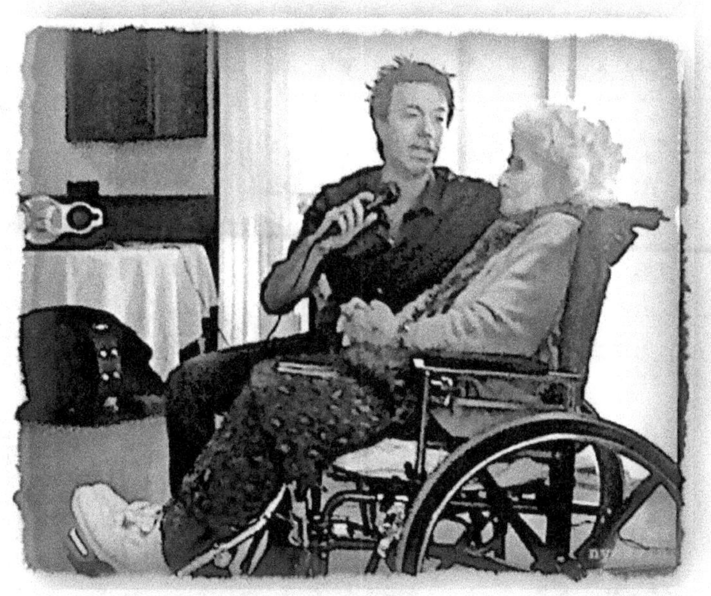

Whenever there were talent shows in her nursing home, she had to sing in them. She looked forward to singing a few of her songs and of course won many contests. I joined Mama in her last talent show and sang with her. It was something I would *never* do when I was growing up. I'd say "Oh no, they're playing guitars and singing those old songs again." Well, the times have changed and singing those old songs became a part of our daily ritual.

The talent show was a week before her transfusion and she was riding high. The

week after the show, again she was in the
hospital getting a transfusion, a definite
low. The roller coaster ride continued...

Back in the hospital, the transfusion
was finally finished while she sang her
favorite song "Some of These Days" for the
umpteenth time imitating Sophie Tucker.
The nurses all spontaneously applauded.
She loved the applause and the attention,
but then again who doesn't? Especially for
someone who *still* wanted to be a singer
when she grew up.

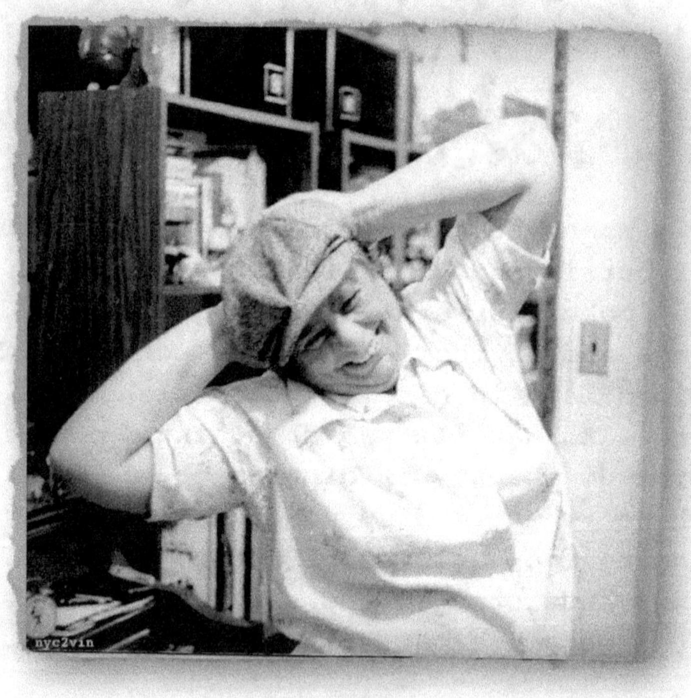

Mama, You're Such An Actress!

Ever since I can remember Mama was an actress. Well, let's put it this way - she always gave me drama. From early on in life, her dream was to be an actress and a singer. The ironic thing is Mama was *always* an actress, she just didn't know it. As far as singing, you couldn't shut her up once she started. Her audience did change over the years. At first it was just family and

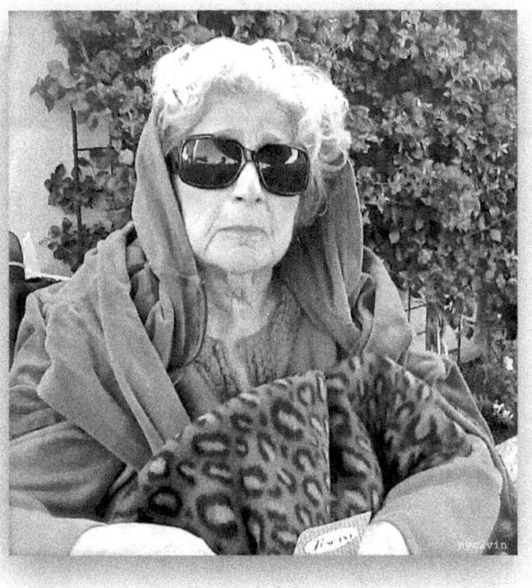

friends, but as time went on, anyone that met her became her audience. In her later years her fans were the nursing home staff, residents, visitors and of course the readers of our blog.

When people ask me if Mama was an actress, I gotta say yes. She was the one who taught me "Never share a spotlight or a microphone". My mother the actress who was always ready for her close up and for anyone who would listen.

      One night as Douglass and I arrived at the nursing home we heard someone ranting rather loudly from down the hall, it was Mama. She was as I liked to call it "Anna-mated". Sometimes we knew what to expect when visiting and decided to play along joining the "Anna with a Z" show, after all she was the star.

Vin: What are you doing acting like that? Are you an actress?

Mama: Of course, I'm a CAREER actress.

Vin: You're a career actress? Since when?

Mama: Since I've been in this damn place. Ya gotta be an actress here.

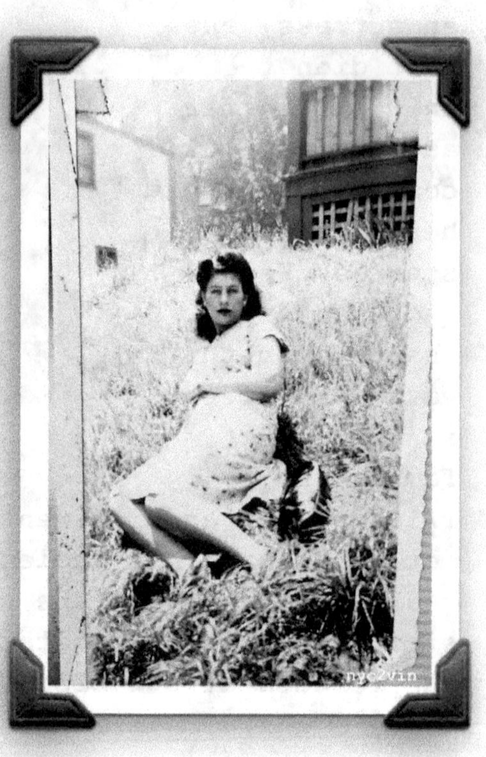

Douglass: What do you mean by that?

Mama: Ya gotta be an actress in this place to get what you want, if you ever wanna get ANYTHING.

Vin: Why do you say that?

Mama: They'd ignore you otherwise. I don't
like to be ignored, so I scream and carry
on. I gotta act like I'm a diva, damn it.
I give them drama! They should give me an
award for the best actress.

   I couldn't have said it better
myself. *"And the Oscar goes to..."*

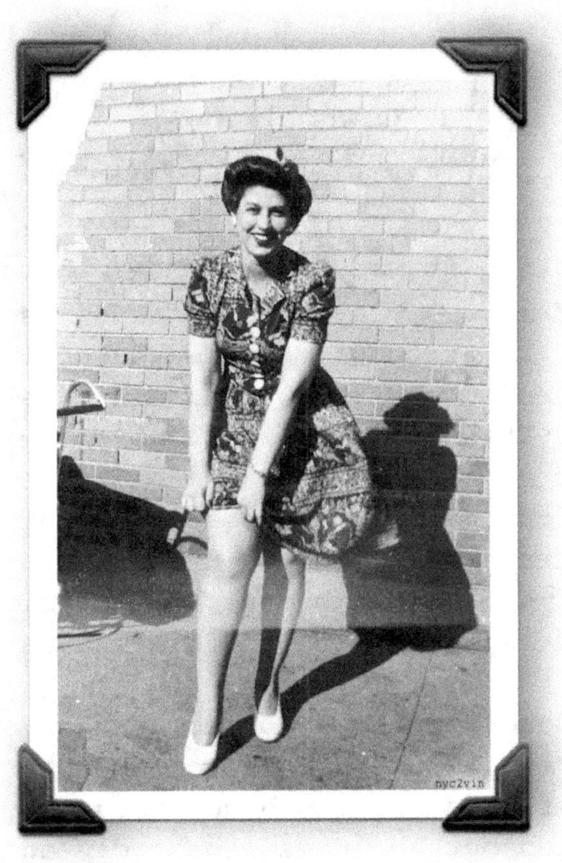

Halloween Scare

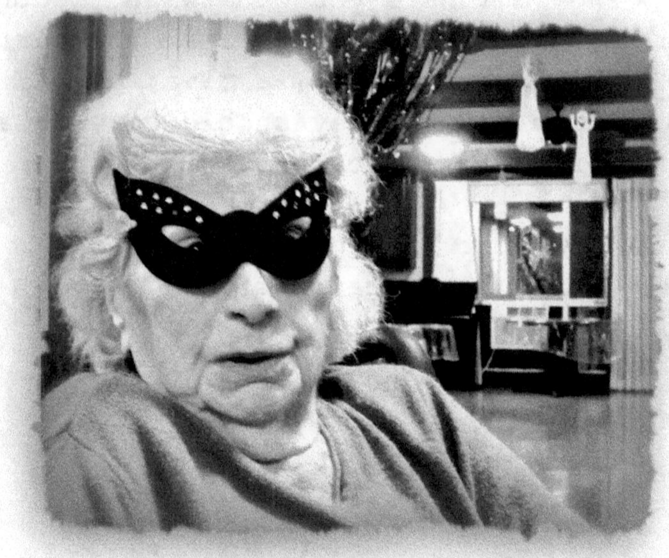

    Since it was Halloween we thought
that Mama was playing a trick on us when
we got to her room. She looked scary. She
was hunched over, drooling and barely
awake. This was definitely NOT a trick. My
mother does not drool. She drops her food,
spits out her food, misses her mouth and
has always been sloppy in the eating
department, but she does NOT drool. I was
scared, I thought this was gonna be it.

    Douglass and I looked at each other,
we were worried. Something was not right
and I felt a warm rush go through my body.
I called out her name repeatedly and
gently tapped her arm as she sat in her

wheelchair with the baseball game on the
television. She wasn't near the TV or even
watching it. This was not typical behavior
for Mama. She loved to watch baseball, no
matter who was playing she always rooted
for the Yankees. She was not responding to
anything at all.

I panicked and overreacted *(another
trait I got from Mama)*. I talked loudly,
trying to get a reaction from her, but she
was still extremely lethargic and did not
react. Douglass wheeled her to the nurses
station and he tried to talk to her as I
ran ahead to the nurse on duty to tell her
what was happening. I wanted to make sure
she didn't have a stroke or had been given
different meds. I asked about her vitals

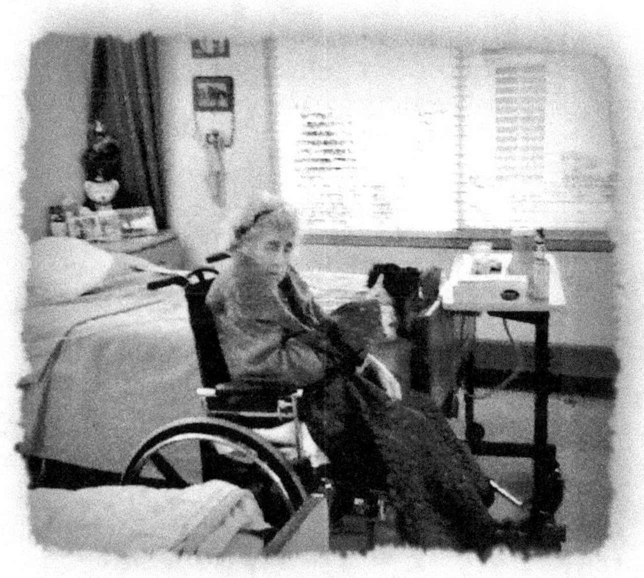

and the nurse said "Everything was fine
when I checked earlier." But I knew that
something was wrong. I wasn't feeling
"fine" about the entire situation and
needed an answer. I was scared for the
first time - really scared. I did not want
Mama to go out with a whimper, drooling
and without a smile or even a song.

We wheeled her into the empty dining
room and tried to feed her some snacks. We
tried to keep her stimulated... but
nothing was working. None of our usual
tricks were working - the cursing, the bad
jokes, the singing, she couldn't even
raise her arms to exercise. I ran back to
the nurses station and insisted that she
check her vitals again and re-evaluate the
situation as Douglass wheeled her back to
her room. Once again all the vitals
appeared fine but I thought it could be
another UTI since she got them so often.
We made sure
she was put
in bed even
though it
was much
earlier than
usual. We
left a few
messages for
the doctor
and stayed

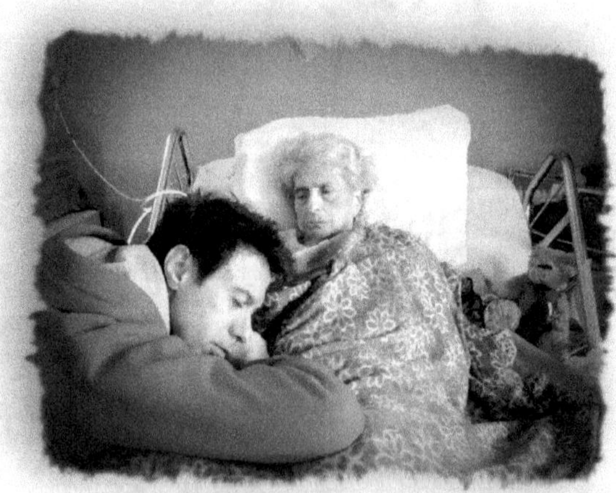

with her for a while waiting for him to
call back. Mama seemed to be resting
comfortably, so we decided to finally go
home and make dinner.

When I called Mama later on that
evening, we both said "I love you" *(as we
always did)* but she sounded weak and was
barely audible. She told me she was saying
her rosary. I told her not to worry and to
think good thoughts.

I kept in touch with the nurses
during the night. I became friendly with
all of them. They were like family and
understood my need to always be on top of
things. So it was no surprise to them that
I insisted they contact the doctor again.
He finally sent an order to run some tests
that I suggested to the nurse earlier.
Douglass and I were still uncomfortable
and anxious for the rest of the night. I
was at a loss and hardly slept at all.
I kept seeing the image of Mama drooling.
I prayed she would be fine in the morning.

The phone woke us up very early in
the morning. My heart was pounding... I
thought the worst. The nurse said that the
tests came back and Mama had pneumonia,
which explained her scary behavior. She
was put on heavy antibiotics immediately.
I'm so glad I was relentless and insisted

on the tests. This scare hit me hard
because the previous week Mama had been
diagnosed with myelodysplasia. Finally we
got an explanation for all the blood
transfusions.

    Myelodysplasia was now more of a
concern than her dementia. In 2012 we were
in the ER three times and the hospital
seven times for transfusions. Mama seemed
to be on deaths door several times and we
were always prepared for the worst. She
would bounce back surprising us every

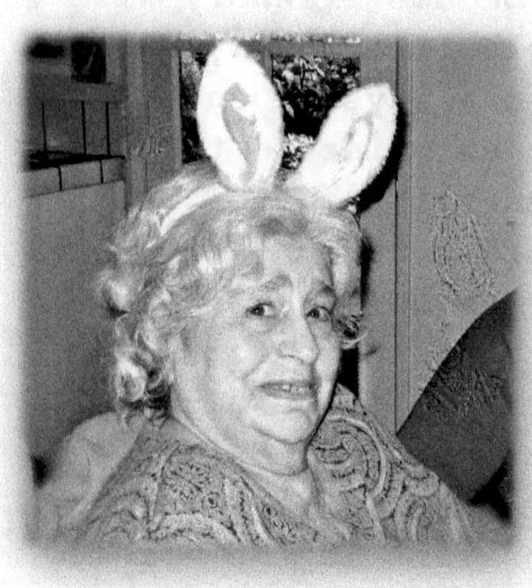

time. We joked
that she was our
"Energizer Bunny".
But with this
latest pneumonia
diagnosis, that
was way too much
Mama Drama even
for me. On that
Halloween night
Mama really did
give us a scare.

Mama Speaks Italian?
Non Capisco!

Every once in a while Mama would sing Italian songs and speak a few words or sentences in Italian. It surprised me because I don't remember hearing much Italian growing up. Sure there were a few curse words or Italian foods, but that was it. We were American and my parents didn't speak Italian - so much for our roots. I remember her pot roast just as much as her lasagna or meatballs.

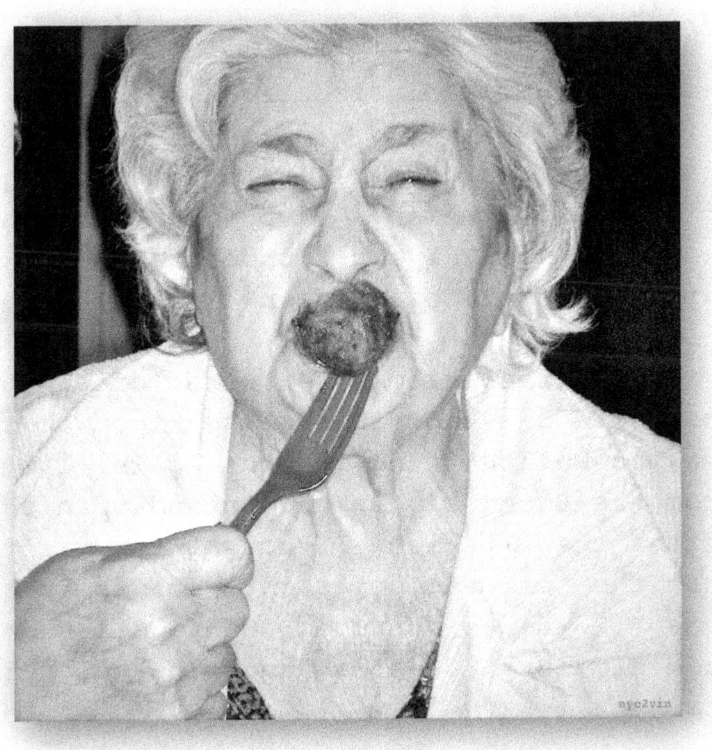

Vin: I've never heard you speak so much
Italian before. This is something new.

Mama: I speak more Italian here than I did
at home. They look at me like I'm crazy
but I'm not crazy, I'm Italian!

Vin: You're not crazy, but I think it's
awfully funny that you've started speaking
all this Italian, especially here. Don't
you?

     She didn't answer, but then started
to sing an old Italian song at the top of
her lungs.

Mama: *"O sole mio, sta'nfronte a te..."*

Vin: Mama, what the hell are you singing?
It's all in Italian. Do you even know what
the words mean? I don't understand, non
capisco. What does it mean?

     She translated a few words of the
song. I don't know if she was right or if
she was bullshitting me once again. I'm
from the Bronx, I can understand Spanish
better than Italian. I thought to myself
what the hell was going on? Who was this
woman? I was so confused. Where did she
suddenly learn to speak and sing all this
Italian?

The staff at the nursing home would occasionally even speak to Mama in some Italian. This was really odd to me because none of them were remotely Italian. It was amusing when Mama played along with them in her version of Italian. I was learning that there were many layers to this thing called dementia. Maybe she recalled it from her early childhood or maybe she even remembered it from a dream. Who knows?

I guess as they say "When in Rome", parla Italiano.

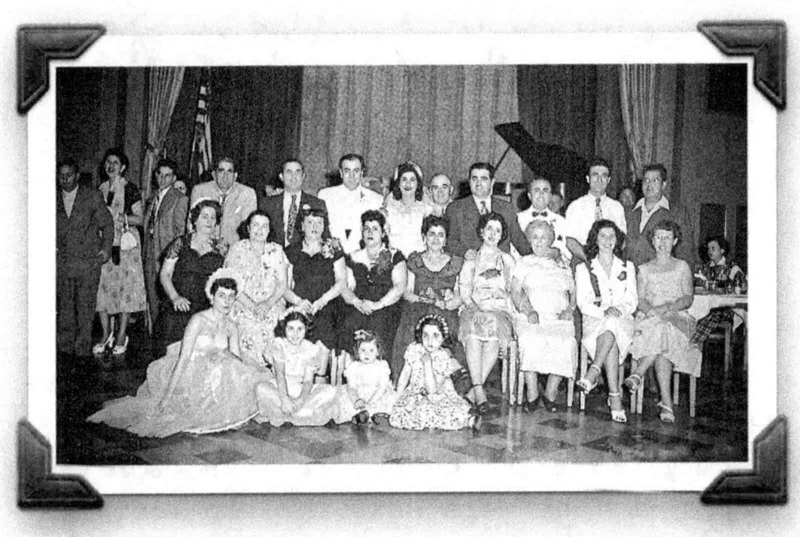

It Could Be Our Last Holiday

Throughout the years Mama would say, "We HAVE to spend the holidays together. Ya never know, it could be our last." I've heard this ever since I can remember, whether it was directed at me or at other family members. Mama's philosophy was simple: Holidays + Family = Happiness!

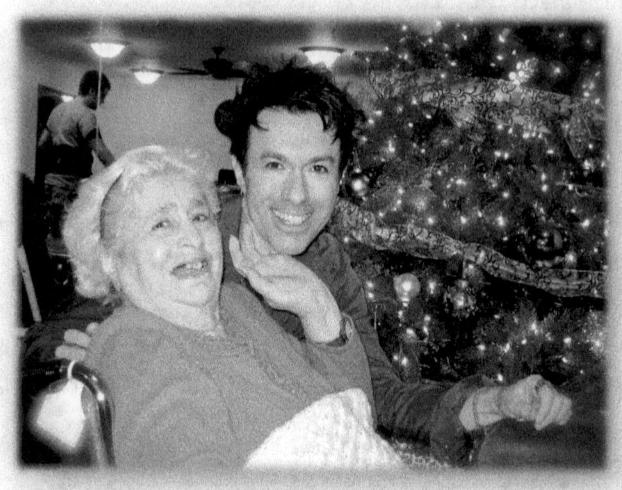

Wow, talk about a guilt trip. It's not only the Catholic guilt or the Italian guilt, but that family was very important to Mama, so I had better be there for the holidays! They were essential to who she was, God forbid I missed one. Once family and friends lost touch or died, her sense of self started to decline along with her health. For me, this proves that we all have the need to be around people and stay connected, especially seniors or those who

have dementia. They tend to be forgotten.
It's something we take for granted.

     What a switch that *I* was now saying
"It could be our last holiday." It's
bizarre that I was thinking and saying
this, but there was a certain amount of
truth to it. Mama's health was getting
worse. The reality was that it could be
our last year to enjoy Christmas together.
Douglass and I were determined to make the
most of it and have a good time, *dammit!*

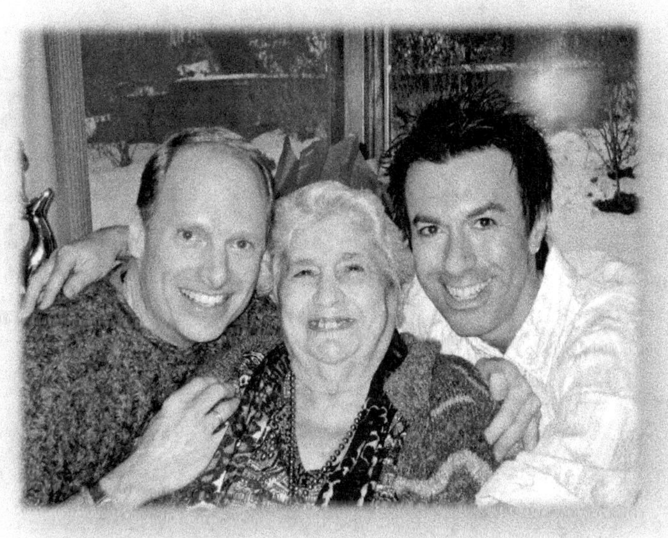

     It killed me knowing that Mama could
die each time Douglass and I went out of
town. We lived with this heavy, dark cloud
hanging over our heads, always getting
darker and hanging lower with her steady
decline - talk about drama!

I know it's good to treat each day as
if it could be our last, and we did most
of the time. But the mix of emotions fast
forwarded, making us feel as if we were
walking on a tightrope and the net was
taken away. I'm not complaining *(well
maybe a little)* but that was how I was
feeling. My emotions were raw and I was
always stressed. I was living on overload.

During her last few years the
holidays consisted of just the three of
us, but it really didn't matter, that's
how it was. We were grateful for whatever
time we had with Mama and we enjoyed it,
because each day was a gift. Another
cliché, but for us it was true now more
than ever. The laughs we shared increased
and that meant the world to Mama. Douglass
and I knew that the end was probably near,
so we planned to make that Christmas the
best we could, because "Ya never know, it
could be our last."

We picked Mama up at the nursing home
and brought her to our place. Whenever we
took her out, there was a checklist. I
laid her clothes out the night before. I'd
call the nurse before we got there to make
sure that she hadn't already eaten, that
her diapers were changed and that she was
ready to go. Taking her over to our place
became increasingly challenging with the

loss of her strength. We had to do all the
work getting her out of the wheelchair and
into the car, then out of the car and into
the wheelchair again. She was not a petite
woman by any means, she was hefty! She'd
yell and scream, then laugh realizing the
ridiculousness of it all. The three of us
were a comical trio, but we did it!

First we toasted with a cocktail and
opened gifts by the tree reminiscing about
Christmas. Mama never cared much about
gifts, she'd never ask for jewelry or any
extravagant things. All she ever wanted
for the holidays was to be with us and of
course to eat her spaghetti and meatballs.

Next came the phone calls. We would
call family and even a few friends from
her old neighborhood. This really made her
light up. She felt connected and close to
her home again.

Finally it was time to wheel her into
our dining room for dinner because of
course she was starving! The table was set
with some of her beautiful old plates that
I had saved for years. It was important
for us to make sure that she was always
surrounded by some familiar things.

For dinner we made a few of her
favorite Italian dishes - cold antipasto,

baked eggplant parmigiana, naturally her spaghetti and meatballs *(which had to be covered with tons of grated parmesan cheese)* and a lot of warm Italian bread.

We continued with coffee, almond cookies and chocolate cake. Then we played cards *(a must for Mama)* even though she'd complain "My hands are killing me. I can't deal these damn cards anymore."

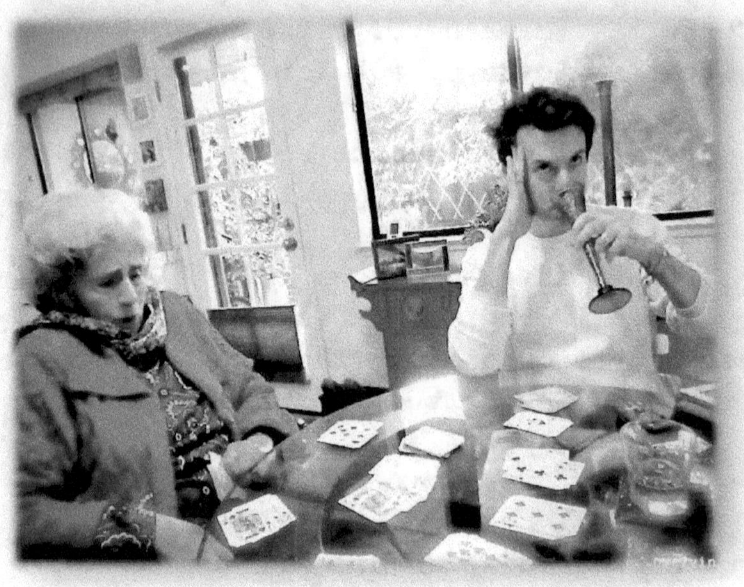

That year, our Christmas was most memorable but bittersweet... *and* it really was our last holiday.

So Happy Together

Mama's Nursing Home was quarantined for nine days due to a flu virus outbreak. It was nine long daze! The few activities scheduled had to be stopped altogether. It left Mama with even *more* time on

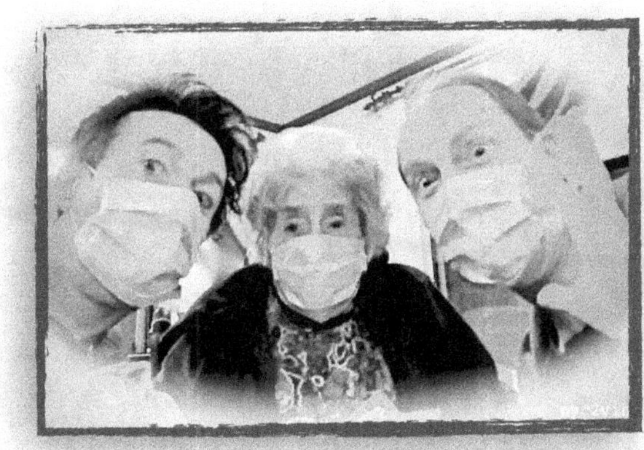

her hands and even *less* time being around others. This did not stop Douglass and me from visiting, even though visitors were "strongly discouraged." We wore masks, just like the staff and residents. It looked and felt odd and Mama hated every minute of wearing a mask...

Mama: I had a crazy dream last night.

Douglass: What did you dream about?

Mama: I dreamt you got married.

Vin: Really? How was the wedding?

Mama: I said to you in my dream, what the hell are you getting married for now? The three of us are already *so* happy together.

     Under my breath I said to Douglass
"We *told* her we got married, she forgot."

Vin: Oh so now you're saying you're *happy*?
Happy? That's a first.

Mama: Yeah I'll be HAPPY when I go home!

     Mama always talked about going home.
Like many with Alzheimer's, she repeatedly
said "I wanna go home, I wanna go home."
I'd tell her she sounded like Dorothy in
"The Wizard of Oz", she'd laugh and change
the subject. I was never sure what she
meant by home. Was it where she was born?
Was it her last apartment? Or was it just
New York? I always got a different answer,
so I never really knew.

Douglass: So Anna, you're not happy?

Mama: Well I'll be happy when I can at
least take this damn mask off and hear
everything that you're saying. Everything
is muffled and I can't breathe. Everybody
is wearing masks in this place, I can't
take this anymore. Do me a favor, please
take this damn mask off me already and
hand me my lipstick.

     Ahhh yes, "Sooo happy together"...

Never Forget

I never lied to Mama, even as a child. Okay, maybe a few times during my teenage years. I have pretty much always told it like it was to both my parents. After Mama was diagnosed with dementia, I may have sugar coated the truth or waited for her reaction but the truth was always told. When family or friends were sick or had died, I'd tell Mama the truth. When she had a health issue, I'd tell Mama the truth. That's just what I did. The truth was important to me.

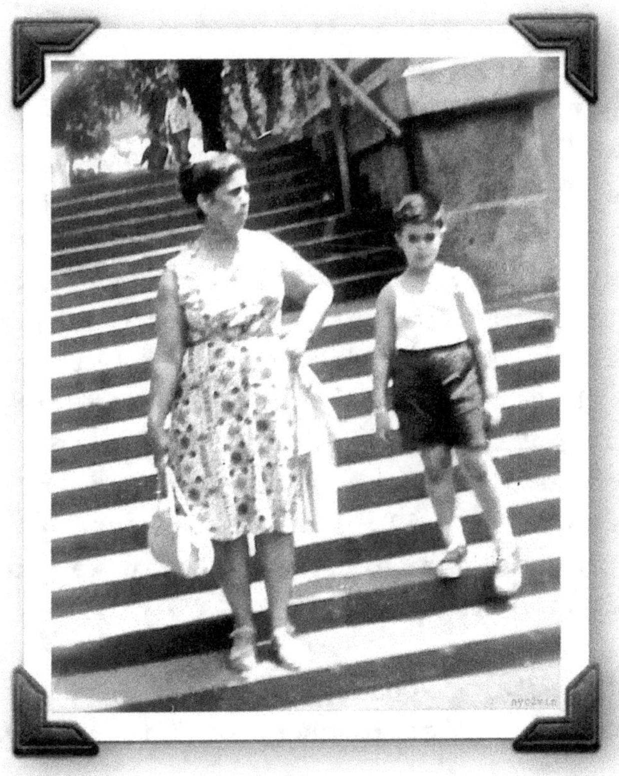

9/11 was no different, I felt Mama
had to be told the truth about the tragedy
that occurred on September 11th. It didn't
matter to me on what level she understood
it, I thought it was important for her to
know about the catastrophe as it was going
on. We lived downtown in the West Village
which was very close to where it happened.
She would be seeing the news nonstop on
television and in the papers and I knew
she would be even more confused. In the
first few days we weren't even allowed to
cross certain streets in our neighborhood
without showing an ID, that's how close we
were to it all.

On that horrendous morning right
after the towers were hit, I ran one block
to the nursing home to check on Mama. I
wanted to make sure that she was okay. I
wheeled her into the middle of the empty
street *(which was usually crowded with
traffic)* to show her a view of what was
happening. We were able to see both towers
from the street and the flames at the top
of the buildings as they burned. We heard
the non-stop sirens. She didn't seem that
interested at all, she just wanted to go
back and eat her pancakes, that was her
main concern.

Douglass and I would wheel Mama down
to the West Side Highway on the Hudson

River almost daily after the towers fell.
We watched the first responders head
downtown as we joined the crowds to cheer
them on. She felt the energy and felt like
she was part of
her city. On
whatever level
she got it, we
were all there
together and
she knew the
truth.

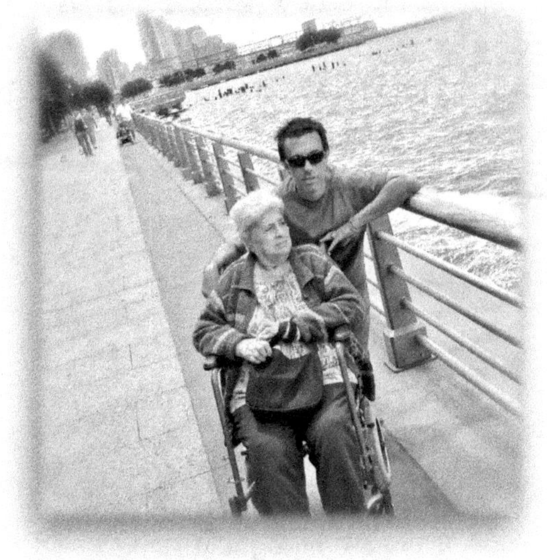

Over the
years I'd ask
Mama what she
remembered
about 9/11. Her
answers varied,
but she usually remembered the feeling
something terrible happened to her city.
Sometimes she remembered the flames or the
empty streets or the cheering crowds. It's
amazing how certain images still remained
in her mind, even with her dementia. It
definitely brings another meaning to the
memorable slogan "Never Forget".

Mama Meets Minnelli

There are other things in your life that you never forget, like when Mama met Liza Minnelli. Meeting Liza epitomizes the New York City experience. It was a chance meeting on the street, no anticipation, just another day in the city.

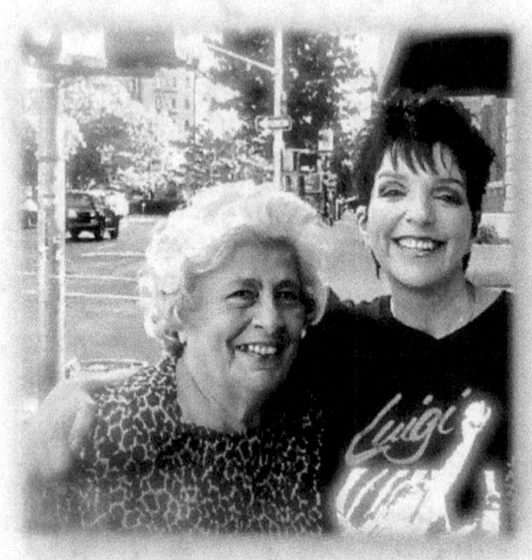

Douglass and I were walking down the street in the West Village to visit Mama at the nursing home. As we passed by an outdoor café, an extremely animated woman caught my eye and I slowed down. Could it be? No way. Is it? OMG, it's Liza Minnelli! I said to Douglass "Slow down, listen to me, there's Liza." He kept walking and looked at me like I was nuts, he didn't believe it was her. I looked at him and said "Mama is finally gonna meet Liza! Go back to the apartment and get the camera" *(we didn't have a camera phone back then).* I ran across 12th Street to get Mama who was sitting on the bench outside the nursing home. I told her "Hurry, get up, come with me and walk to the corner - Mama, you're finally gonna meet Liza Minnelli." I never saw Mama walk so fast with her walker. Douglass now had the camera and the three of us tried to act casual as we strolled by the restaurant. Then we realized that Liza was now standing directly in front of us on the sidewalk smoking a cigarette. Oh my God, "Vin with a Z" was taking "Anna with a Z" to meet "Liza with a Z". We were totally Z'd to the max!

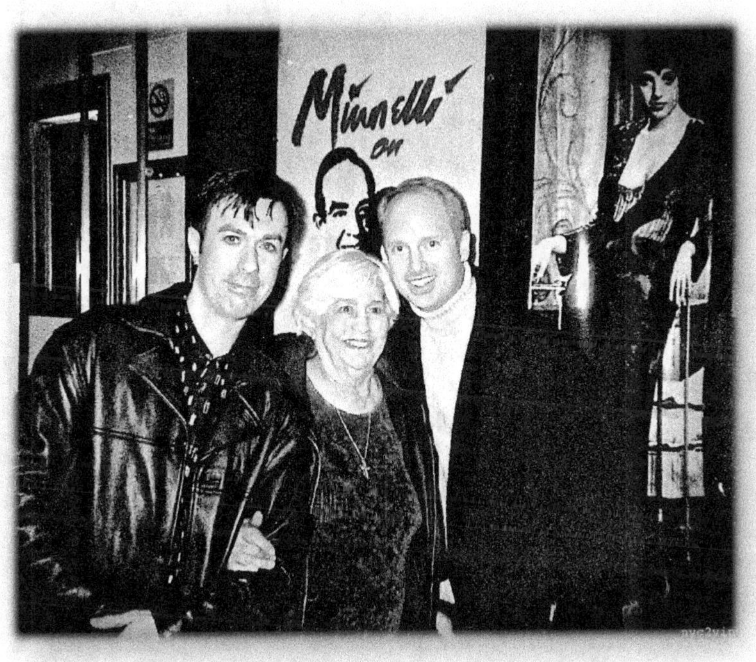

I lightly tapped Liza on her shoulder and introduced the three of us. She was very gracious and warm, acting more like

an old friend than a celebrity. Insisting
on taking a few pictures with us, she
hugged us all repeatedly and then signed
an autograph for Mama. Liza kept talking
and talking as if we had known her for
years, just like you would expect her to
do. She even joked with me, calling
me "Daddy" since my name is Vincent just
like her father, Vincente Minnelli, who
also suffered with Alzheimer's.

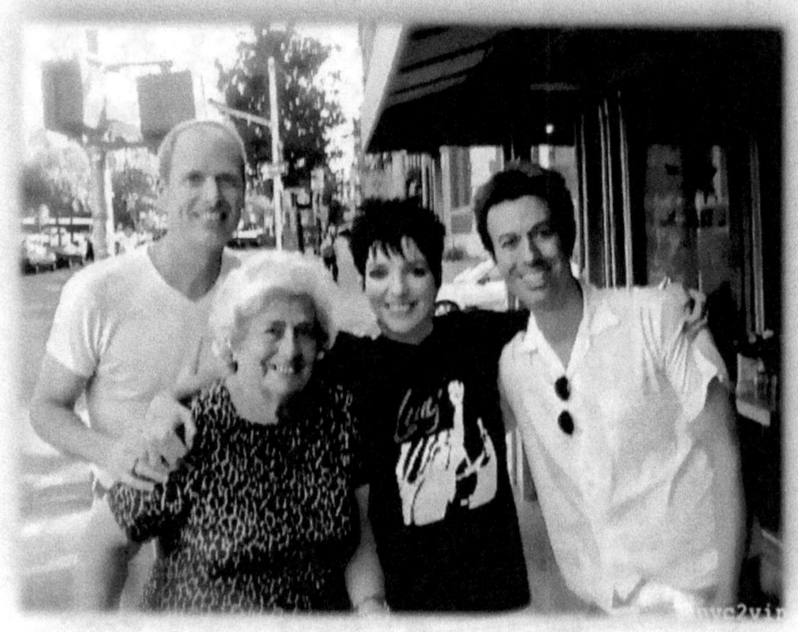

     Liza made our day, but even more
importantly she made Mama's day. It was a
most memorable meeting, especially Iy for
Mama. She loved Liza and went to many of
her shows with us. She always kept the
photo of the four of us by her bedside in

the nursing home. Mama never forgot that day and would proudly tell people about the time she met Liza Minnelli. When we ran into Liza a few years later, I told her about that day and how much it meant to Mama. She was very touched and said "Oh baby, I'm so glad."

I'll be eternally grateful to Liza for being so giving to the three of us on the street that day and leaving Mama with a lasting memory.

Mama met Minnelli and it meant the world to her. She would tell the story again and again and again. To quote a song from Vincente Minnelli's classic MGM film "Gigi"... *"Ah yes, I remember it well."* And so did Mama!

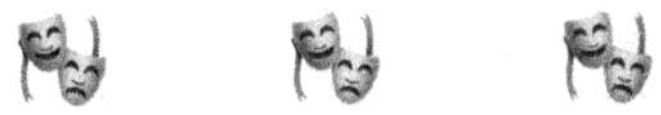

Goodnight My Love

I felt bad that Douglass and I couldn't be back in time for our nightly visit with Mama. When Mama had the nurse call me (*for the third time*) I reminded her *again* that we wouldn't be seeing her that night because it had been a crazy day and we still weren't even home yet. She sighed but then her tone became lighter as she started to sing me a song from one of her favorite MGM stars, Shirley Temple.

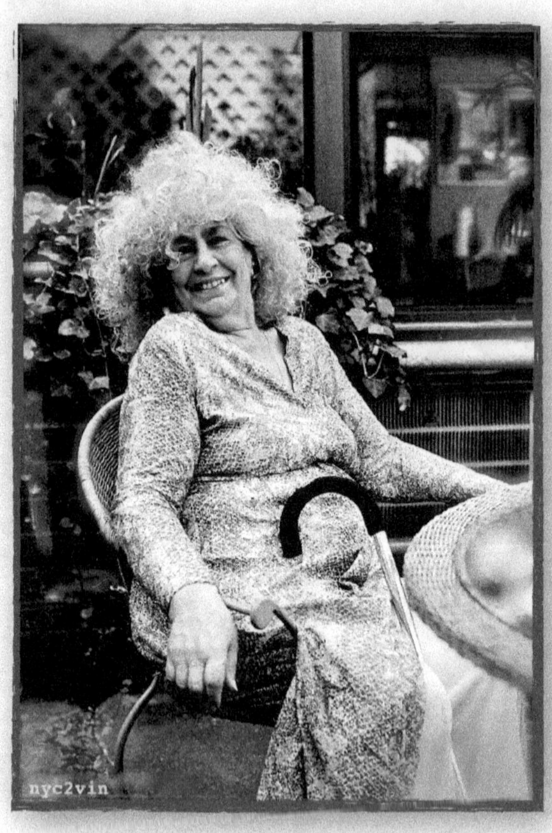

Mama: *"Goodnight my love, your mommy is kneeling beside you. Goodnight my love, to dreamland the sandman will guide you. Come now you sleepy head, close your eyes go to bed. My precious sleepyhead, you mustn't play peek-a-boo..."*

This went on for quite a while. How the hell did she remember all those words? Proof again that music stays in your memory the longest. It was odd that even over the phone she could sense that I had a stressful day. I listened to her as she finished the song.

Vin: Thanks Ma, that was a very sweet song. Sorry we can't see you tonight, but we'll see you tomorrow night. Thanks for the song. I love you.

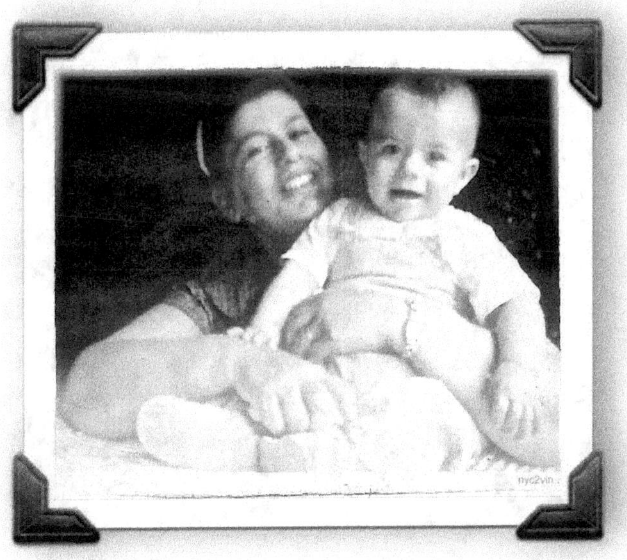

Mama: Thank you. I love you too, my son.

Vin: Goodnight Mama.

Mama: Goodnight dear. You're going to see
me tomorrow, *right?*

Vin: Yes, of course Ma. By the way, did
you have any visitors today? (*I knew that
our friend had stopped by earlier with her
dog for some pet therapy.*)

Mama: No, no one stopped by today.

Vin: Are you sure?

Mama: *(After a long pause)* Oh yeah, a nice
lady with a dog was here. You know I
always had dogs growing up. I miss them.
But I love her puppy, she makes me forget.

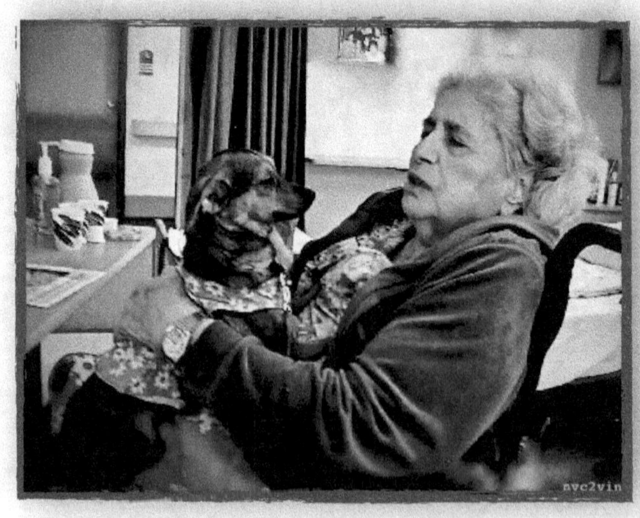

Vin: **Maybe you shouldn't love the puppy so much, if it makes you forget.**

Mama: **What are you talking about?**

Vin: **I'm talking about the puppy. What are you talking about?**

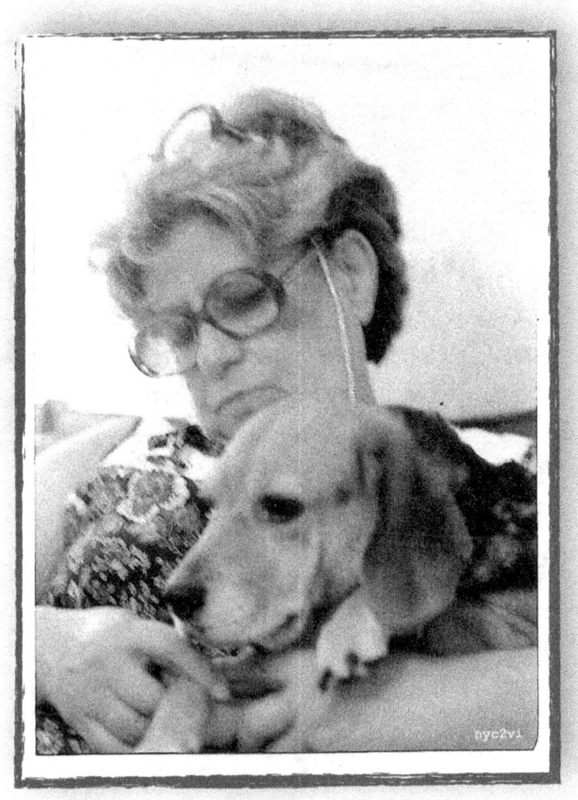

Mama: **I dunno, I forgot. I guess the puppy made me forget.**

Vin: **Forget what?** *(Pushing her buttons and egging her on)*

Mama: Vincent you're driving me crazy. I love the damn puppy and that's that.

Vin: That's what?

Mama: Oh forget it, I already did. I wish I could just forget I'm in this place.

Vin: So you're complaining about the place again. Well, look at the bright side, at least you had some company today. I'm glad you did.

Mama: Me too. Now just stay home tonight and get some sleep. I'll see you tomorrow.

I knew Mama was getting weaker and I wasn't sure how many songs she had left in her. We said goodnight once again and I sang a few lines of the song...

"*Come now you sleepy head, close your eyes go to bed. Goodnight my love.*"

Do You Have My Number?

The phone rang earlier than usual. It was the nursing home calling and naturally I thought the worst. I never knew what was coming next when the nursing home called, that's why I didn't shut off my phone. I had it on 24/7 just in case. What could be going on this time? Was everything all right? My heart began to race as I took a few deep breaths and picked up my phone...

Mama: Hello, is this Vincent?

Vin: Hello Ma, of course it's me. It's early in the morning. Are you okay?

Mama: Oh yeah, I'm just fine. Do you have my phone number? I called because I wanna make sure that you have my phone number.

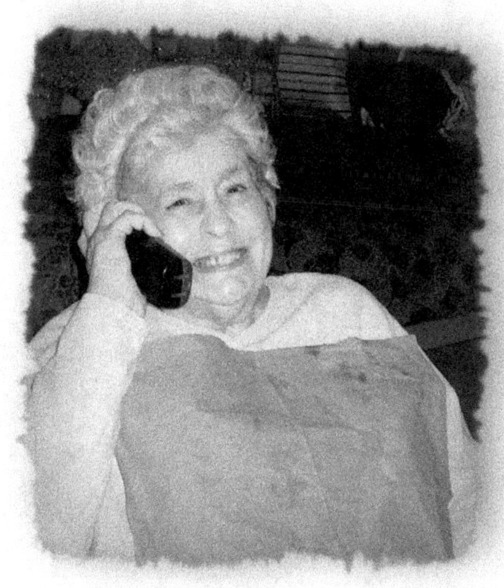

Vin: Yes, of course I have your number. It's the same number you've had, it hasn't changed.

Mama: Okay, and you know where I am don't you? You have my address? I'm at the home.

Vin: Yes I know where you are, you're in
the nursing home a few blocks away.

Mama: Will I be seeing you later?

Vin: Yes Ma. I'll be seeing you after your
dinner just like every night.

Mama: Well then, be careful coming over
and watch the street when you cross. It's
very dangerous out there. Ohhh thank God,
the food is finally here. I gotta go, I
gotta eat now! I'm starving. I hope it's
something good. You know they serve a lot
of crap in here. Ohhh goodie, looks like
pancakes. Bye bye dear, I gotta go now.

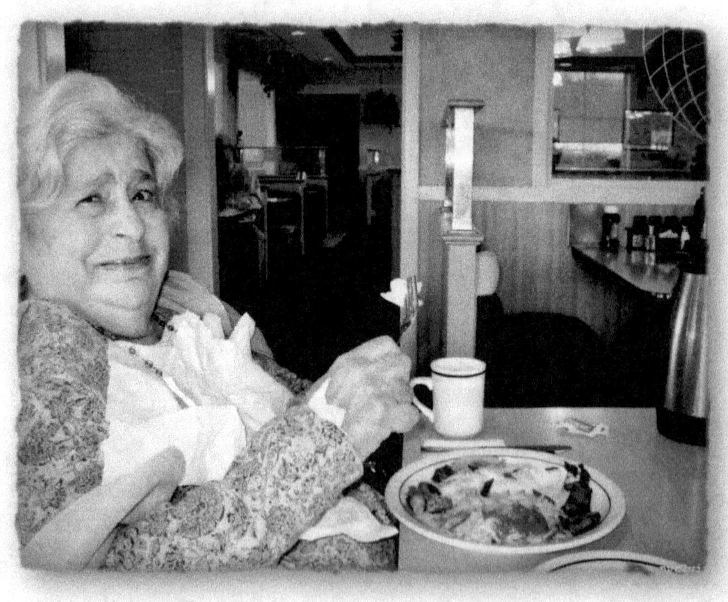

Over The Rainbow

When is the right time to have "the talk"? No, not the talk you had with your parents about the birds and the bees. I could only imagine how difficult that talk is for many parents. The talk I mean is the one you have with your aging parents about letting go and dying. The final talk when it's obvious that the end is near.

When is it too early? It's obvious when it's too late! But then once you say it, you can't undo it. There's no erase button. It's all about timing.

Will Mama understand? Will she get it? Will she ignore it or break out into song so she didn't have to deal with it once again?

Mama and I had "the talk" many times during her last few months but I was never quite sure if she fully understood it. How many times can you say goodbye to a loved one? The answer for me was many times and it *never* got easier.

Some days I would very bluntly say "Mama if you wanna die, then just die... it's okay." While on other days I'd say things that "should" be said to comfort her and to help her follow the yellow

brick road and finally be able to go over
the rainbow.

        We said our goodbyes over and over.
We strolled down memory lane so many times
that it needed repaving. We talked about
going to the light so often, that we
needed a new lightbulb. We went thru the
entire list of people she missed and the
names just kept coming. I constantly
assured her that she would see them all
again and finally be with her brothers,
sisters, family and friends.

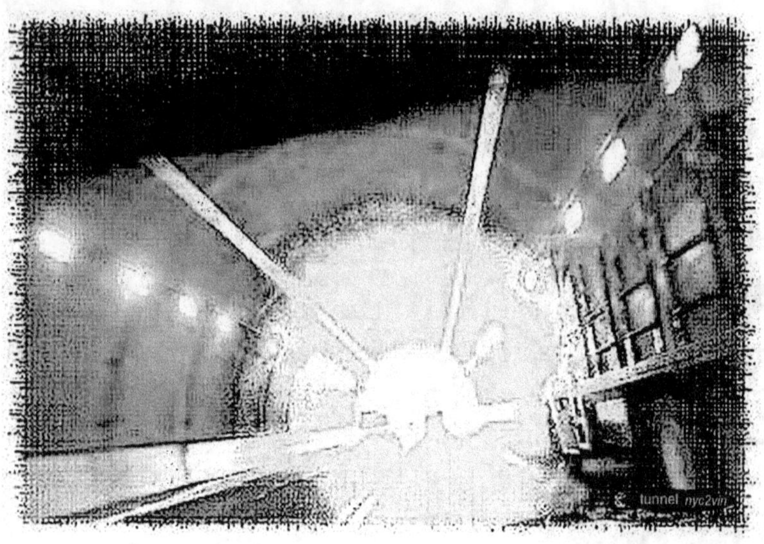

        I had to make sure that she knew she
didn't have to worry about me any longer.
That was a very difficult one since she
was always so overprotective. I knew it
wouldn't be easy for her to finally let go

of her son. I'd be fine, I constantly had
to reassure her of this. I reminded her
that I had Douglass, family and friends
that would be there for me. I told her I
was a tough cookie just like her which
always brought a smile to her face. I'd
say it's okay to let go... "Let go, go
towards the light." It seemed so cliché
but no one ever said it didn't work.

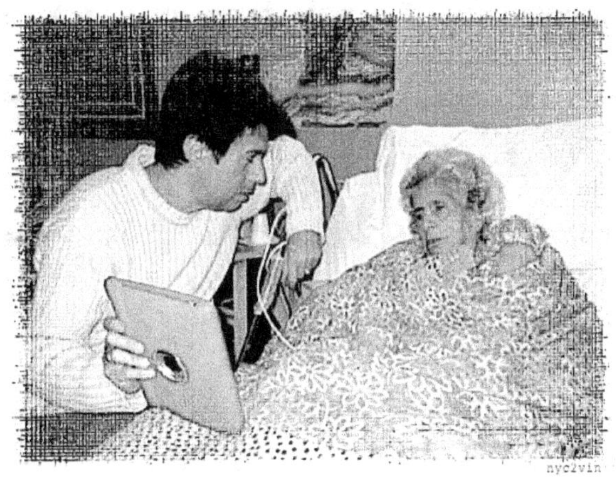

But the question was would *I* be ready
to let go? Her final curtain forced me to
face my mortality and question who would
be *my* advocate in the end? Before this, I
knew I'd survive anything because my job
was to take care of Mama, so I HAD to
survive. But what happens now? I was sad,
scared and very vulnerable.

Since moving to California, Mama was
my only true friend, I didn't have many

friends there. It's odd, but it was the
truth. We saw each other and spoke on the
phone everyday. We'd talk about anything
and everything. I would be losing my best
friend and I wouldn't know what to do...
and then that day came.

I consider myself extremely lucky to
have had "the talk" with my parents and I
know that it made it easier for both of
them to let go. I know it made it easier
for me. I remember being in the hospice
with my father and asking all the family
to leave the room so I could have the talk
with him. I don't know how I gathered the
strength or found the words, but I did.
The last time I had the talk with Mama,
it must have sunk in and she was ready for
her next act. Douglass and I were there
with her and kept playing her favorite
songs over and over. Once again music got
us through. It's ironic that she left us
while listening to the lyrics *"If happy
little bluebirds fly beyond the rainbow
why, oh why, can't I?"* Mama always knew
how to make an exit!

The most difficult part for me was my
transition of life without Mama. Since
then I take it day by day and cherish our
many memories. Unlike Mama, I can clearly
recall most of them. I continued telling
our story just like she wanted me to do by

writing about her and sharing our photos. The pictures would always spark her memory and make her feel better just like music did. She really got a kick out of looking at them - the old *and* the new. Now they're doing the same thing for me.

Mama didn't want to be forgotten, but anyone who met her or read about her could never forget her and her love of life. She was always one helluva colorful character.

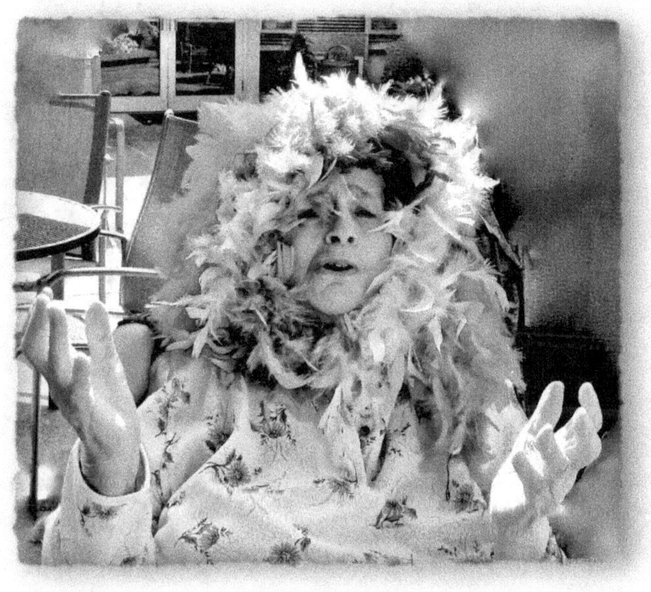

Saying It Out Loud

By now you must know that I believe in being honest, sometimes a little too honest, but that's just me. It took me a long time to fully accept the fact that Mama died... there, I said it out loud. Mama died.

We all assumed that Mama would die from dementia but instead myelodysplasia crept into our lives. We knew nothing about it, only that it's a form of leukemia that affected Robin Roberts of ABC News at that 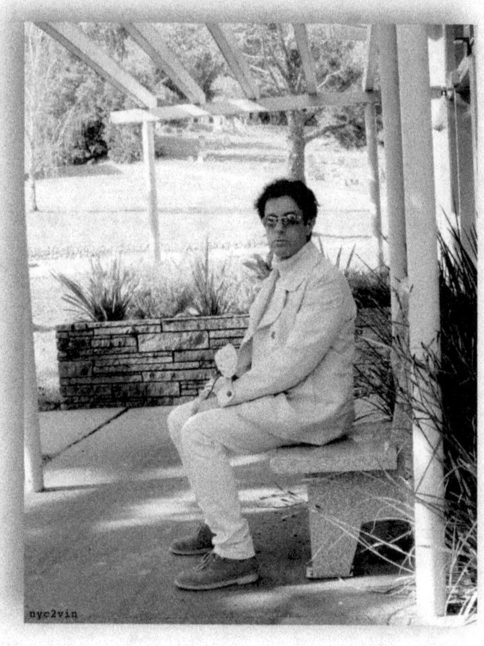

time. She was much younger and fortunate to find a bone marrow donor. Mama was too old for that and chemo was not an option at her age either. We only had one other alternative, blood transfusions. On those "Transfusion Confusion Daze" Mama would moan, "Why do I have to go to the hospital again? And why do I need more of this damn blood? I have enough of my own. When are

we gonna get the hell outta here? I'm
starving and my ass is killing me!"

I avoided saying that Mama was dead
for quite a while. I wasn't sure how to
handle it but I needed to say it out loud.
As you know by now Douglass and I were her
caregivers for over thirteen years and
were with her almost everyday. The entire
experience seems so surreal now. How did
we ever do it? This was even before there
was much help available for caregivers. We
didn't follow the rules, we just did what
came naturally.

For a long
time after she
died, we still
checked the clock
thinking it was
time to be at the
nursing home. And
I still checked
the phone for her
daily long winded
messages. It was
our routine for
so many years

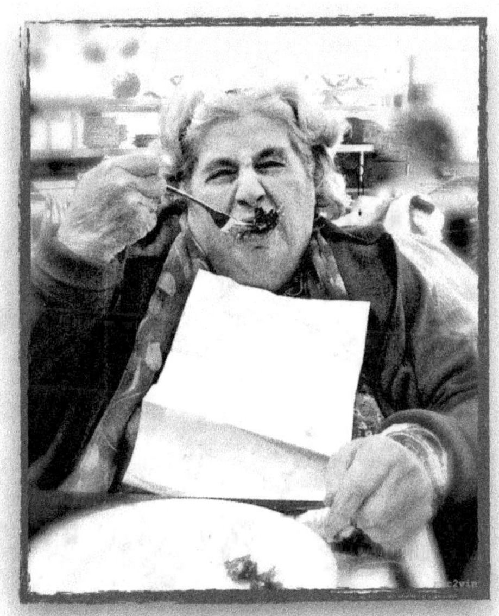

that it became second nature. We still
thought it was time to be singing, playing
cards, exercising or cursing with her to
make her laugh. But Mama was gone and no
longer here.

I promised Mama that we'd continue
with our book. She loved performing and
being interviewed. She enjoyed watching
the videos we took of her and sang along
with them. She was always ready to put on
a costume and pose for photos and then
laughed looking at them. If we didn't take
any photos she'd say "Why the hell aren't
you taking my picture tonight?" We knew it
gave her another reason to keep going. The
book developed into a play which premiered
at The Fringe Festival as "Some Of These
Daze". Mama was always a larger than life
character so it was only fitting that her
story belonged on the stage.

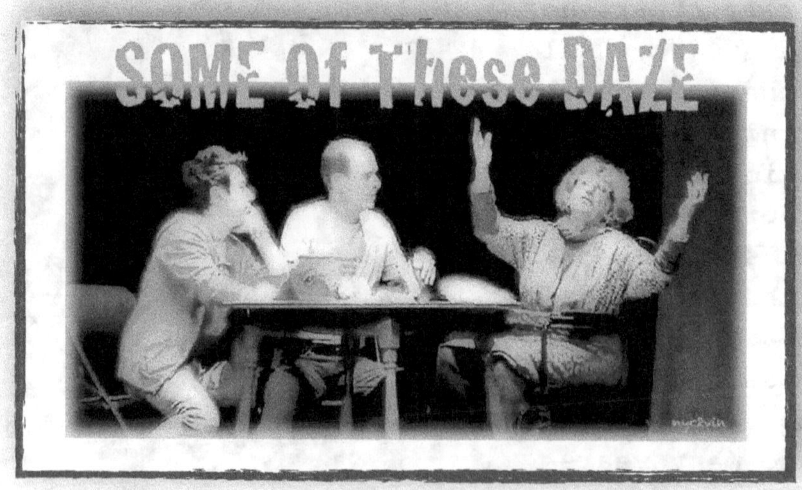

Douglass and I are still advocates
for Alzheimers, dementia, myelodysplasia
and Women's Heart Disease, all of which
affected Mama. We've continued to bring

awareness to these diseases and do what we can through social media.

Mama may have left her physical body which was failing her, but her energy is still very much alive. Her spirit, sense of humor, neurosis *and* drama all still live through me. Strange as it sounds, not a day goes by I don't feel her presence. We always had a strong bond and she'll continue to be our "Dementia-Mama-Drama".

The fact that the three of us could still laugh and sing when everything else around us seemed unbearable was pretty damn incredible. It was proof that love can get you through. And like Mama always sang in "Some of These Days" her signature tune *"You're gonna miss your big fat mama, some of these days."*

Mama, you are loved, you are missed and you are finally a star!

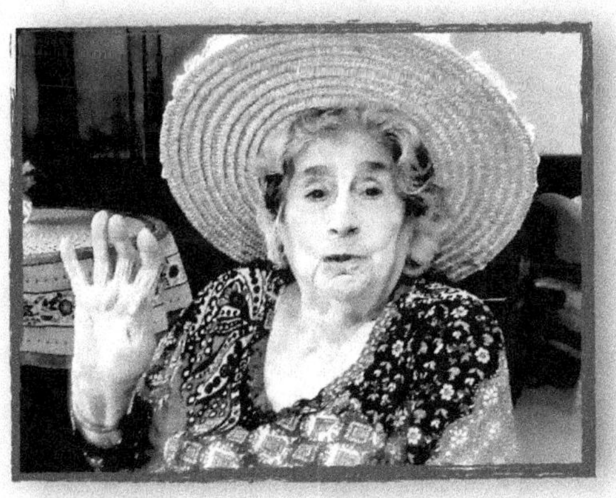

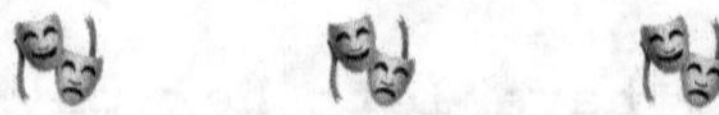

These organizations have been a part of our ride with *Dementia-Mama-Drama*. We have continued to support them and we encourage you to do the same.

Alzheimer's Los Angeles
alzheimersla.org

Leeza's Care Connection
leezascareconnection.org

The Dawn Method
thedawnmethod.com

Alzheimer's Association
alz.org

MDS Foundation
mds-foundation.org

Women's Heart Alliance
womensheartalliance.org

About The Author

Vincent Zappacosta has been a writer and photographer ever since he was a little boy back in Catholic school. His professional background includes graphic design, theatre and yoga.

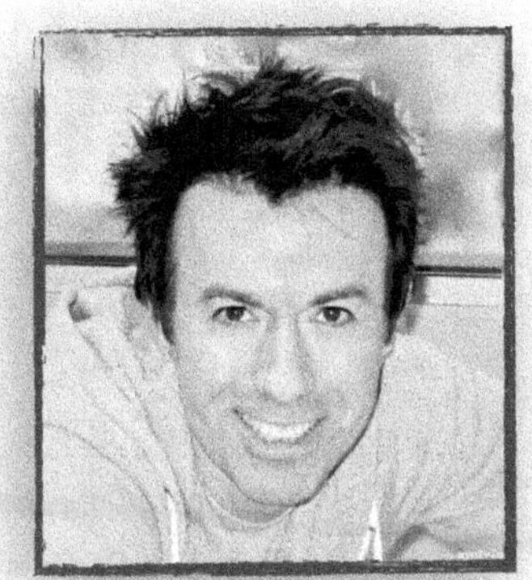

His writings as a caregiver and a strong advocate for dementia and **Alzheimer's** have been published by several leading Alzheimer's organizations. He has received national awards for his graphic design but still has room on his shelf for more.

Vincent and Douglass Christensen, his husband, continue work on "Some Of These Daze" the script based on their experiences as caregivers for Mama. She will finally be on the stage and screen where she belongs.

Social Media Links

Dementia-Mama-Drama
BLOG: Dementia-Mama-Drama.com
TWITTER: Dementia Mama
FACEBOOK: Dementia.Mama.Drama
INSTAGRAM: Dementia-Mama-Drama

Some Of These Daze
FACEBOOK: Some Of These Daze

Mama's Fans

"She was an inspiration for so many, making us laugh and cry. Thank you for sharing her story and for showing people the joy and struggles of being a caregiver."
> ~ Patty Guinto, Alzheimer's Association

"Always honest, real and inspiring posts from Dementia-Mama-Drama. I've enjoyed following the journey. Thanks for sharing and baring your soul, telling the story and making it count."
> ~ Leeza Gibbons, Leeza's Care Connection

"As a clinician, this is a MUST-READ for all. The author shares a glimpse into how dementia affected Mama and her journey with her son, son-in-law and life in general. As the reader, we're able to feel the trials and tribulations the family ventured through together. You will find yourself laughing, crying sometimes out of sadness and other times out of pure joy."
> ~ Nettie Harper, Inspired Memory Care

"Despite the heavy subject matter, it's handled with grace and humor bringing an unexpected levity to the struggles of caregiving. A touching relatable story that would serve anyone dealing with dementia. A must-read."
> ~ Valma Da Silva, Gentle Wave Services

"The most important ingredients in caregiving, heart and humor are abundant in this book. A short uplifting read that will remind you to sprinkle these ingredients generously in your own life tasks."
> ~ Gerrda Greiner-Focardi, LITA Marin

"A warm, funny, ultimately hopeful look at caring for a parent. I related to many of the challenges chronicled, having lost family to Alzheimer's. The author put into words many of the emotions that I felt. A great resource for families dealing with the same situation. The photos and stories managed to beautifully tie the present and past together."
> ~ Stacey Nerdin

"The book is a quick read that tells the story of a fun loving woman and the son she adores. They feed off each other with humor and love. Thank you for telling Mama's story with grace, humor and a dose of reality."
> ~ Kelly Abbatantuono

"The book pulls back the curtain and offers a candid, unapologetic look at the ups and downs caregivers and patients face every hour of every day in the world of dementia. It is a testament to what the power of unconditional love, relentless determination and total commitment can do."
> ~ William Babb

Mama's Prayer Card

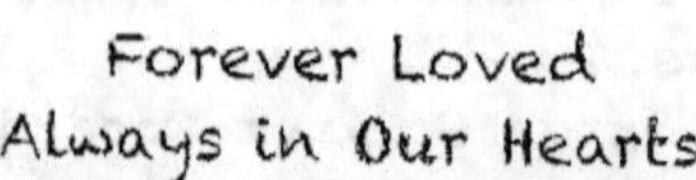

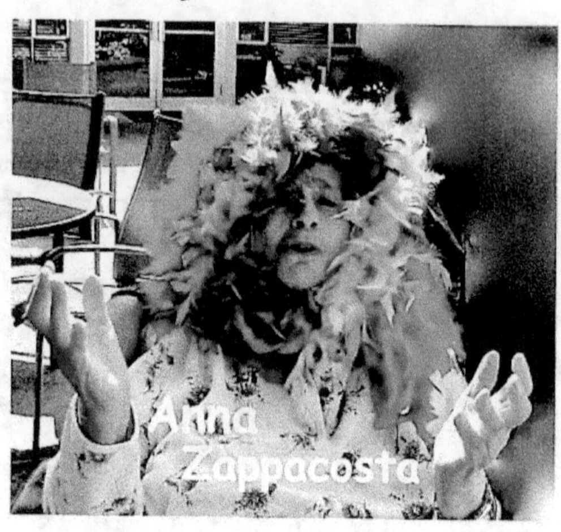

Anna's Daily Prayers...

"Holy Mary Mother of God,
Chase the Chickens
'Round the Yard."

"Let's Play Cards Already"

"I Want Spaghetti & Meatballs"

"I Wanna Go Home"

"You're Gonna Miss Your Big
Fat Mama, Some of These Days"

Notes:

www.ingramcontent.com/pod-product-compliance
Lightning Source LLC
Chambersburg PA
CBHW070849250726
48662CB00003B/1437